Serono Symposia, USA
Norwell, Massachusetts

## PROCEEDINGS IN THE SERONO SYMPOSIA, USA SERIES

*OVARIAN CELL INTERACTIONS: Genes to Physiology*
Edited by Aaron J.W. Hsueh and David W. Schomberg

*IN VITRO FERTILIZATION AND EMBRYO TRANSFER IN PRIMATES*
Edited by Don P. Wolf, Richard L. Stouffer, and Robert M. Brenner

*CELL BIOLOGY AND BIOTECHNOLOGY: Novel Approaches to Increased Cellular Productivity*
Edited by Melvin S. Oka and Randall G. Rupp

*PREIMPLANTATION EMBRYO DEVELOPMENT*
Edited by Barry D. Bavister

*MOLECULAR BASIS OF REPRODUCTIVE ENDOCRINOLOGY*
Edited by Peter C.K. Leung, Aaron J.W. Hsueh, and Henry G. Friesen

*MODES OF ACTION OF GnRH AND GnRH ANALOGS*
Edited by William F. Crowley, Jr., and P. Michael Conn

*FOLLICLE STIMULATING HORMONE: Regulation of Secretion and Molecular Mechanisms of Action*
Edited by Mary Hunzicker-Dunn and Neena B. Schwartz

*SIGNALING MECHANISMS AND GENE EXPRESSION IN THE OVARY*
Edited by Geula Gibori

*GROWTH FACTORS IN REPRODUCTION*
Edited by David W. Schomberg

*UTERINE CONTRACTILITY: Mechanisms of Control*
Edited by Robert E. Garfield

*NEUROENDOCRINE REGULATION OF REPRODUCTION*
Edited by Samuel S.C. Yen and Wylie W. Vale

*FERTILIZATION IN MAMMALS*
Edited by Barry D. Bavister, Jim Cummins, and Eduardo R.S. Roldan

*GAMETE PHYSIOLOGY*
Edited by Ricardo H. Asch, Jose P. Balmaceda, and Ian Johnston

*GLYCOPROTEIN HORMONES: Structure, Synthesis, and Biologic Function*
Edited by William W. Chin and Irving Boime

*THE MENOPAUSE: Biological and Clinical Consequences of Ovarian Failure: Evaluation and Management*
Edited by Stanley G. Korenman

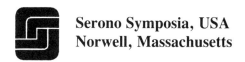

Serono Symposia, USA
Norwell, Massachusetts

Aaron J.W. Hsueh   David W. Schomberg
Editors

# Ovarian Cell Interactions
## Genes to Physiology

With 61 Figures

Springer-Verlag
New York Berlin Heidelberg London Paris
Tokyo Hong Kong Barcelona Budapest

Aaron J.W. Hsueh, Ph.D.
Department of Obstetrics and
 Gynecology
Division of Reproductive Biology
Stanford University Medical Center
Stanford, CA 94305
USA

David W. Schomberg, Ph.D.
Department of Obstetrics and
 Gynecology
Division of Reproductive Biology
Duke University Medical Center
Durham, NC 27710
USA

Proceedings of the Ninth Ovarian Workshop on Ovarian Cell Interactions: Genes to Physiology, sponsored by Serono Symposia, USA, held July 9 to 11, 1992, in Chapel Hill, North Carolina.

For information on previous volumes, please contact Serono Symposia, USA.

Library of Congress Cataloging-in-Publication Data
Ovarian cell interactions: genes to physiology/Aaron J.W. Hsueh,
 David W. Schomberg, editors.—1st ed.
   p. cm.
  "Serono Symposia, USA."
  "Ninth Ovarian Workshop on Ovarian Cell Interactions: Genes to Physiology was held at the University of North Carolina–Chapel Hill in 1992"—Pref.
  Includes bibliographical references and index.
  ISBN 0-387-94052-9 (acid-free paper)
  1. Ovaries—Physiology—Congresses.  2. Ovaries—Molecular aspects—Congresses.  I. Hsueh, Aaron J.W.  II. Schomberg, David W.
III. Ovarian Workshop on Ovarian Cell Interactions: Genes to Physiology (1992: University of North Carolina–Chapel Hill)
QP261.0846  1993
599'.033—dc20                                                           93-27845

Printed on acid-free paper.

© 1993 Springer-Verlag New York, Inc.
All rights reserved. This work may not be translated or copied in whole or in part without the written permission of the publisher (Springer-Verlag New York, Inc., 175 Fifth Avenue, New York, NY 10010, USA), except for brief excerpts in connection with reviews or scholarly analysis. Use in connection with any form of information storage and retrieval, electronic adaptation, computer software, or by similar or dissimilar methodology now known or hereafter developed is forbidden.
The use of general descriptive names, trade names, trademarks, etc., in this publication, even if the former are not especially identified, is not to be taken as a sign that such names, as understood by the Trade Marks and Merchandise Marks Act, may accordingly be used freely by anyone.
While the advice and information in this book are believed to be true and accurate at the date of going to press, neither the authors, nor the editors, nor the publisher, nor Serono Symposia, USA, nor Serono Laboratories, Inc., can accept any legal responsibility for any errors or omissions that may be made. The publisher makes no warranty, expressed or implied, with respect to the material contained herein.
Permission to photocopy for internal or personal use, or the internal or personal use of specific clients, is granted by Springer-Verlag New York, Inc., for libraries registered with the Copyright Clearance Center (CCC), provided that the base fee of $5.00 per copy, plus $0.20 per page is paid directly to CCC, 21 Congress Street, Salem, MA 01970, USA. Special requests should be addressed directly to Springer-Verlag New York, Inc., 175 Fifth Avenue, New York, NY 10010, USA.

Production coordinated by Marilyn Morrison and managed by Francine McNeill; manufacturing supervised by Jacqui Ashri.
Typeset by Best-set Typesetter Ltd., Hong Kong.
Printed and bound by Edwards Brothers, Inc., Ann Arbor, MI.

Printed in the United States of America.

9 8 7 6 5 4 3 2 1

ISBN 0-387-94052-9 Springer-Verlag New York Berlin Heidelberg
ISBN 3-540-94052-9 Springer-Verlag Berlin Heidelberg New York

# NINTH OVARIAN WORKSHOP ON OVARIAN CELL INTERACTIONS: GENES TO PHYSIOLOGY

**Ovarian Workshop Board**

>Aaron J.W. Hsueh, Ph.D., Chairman
>Stanford, California
>
>David W. Schomberg, Ph.D., Chairman
>Durham, North Carolina
>
>Eli Adashi, M.D.
>Baltimore, Maryland
>
>Jennifer Dorrington, Ph.D.
>Toronto, Ontario
>
>John Eppig, Ph.D.
>Bar Harbor, Maine
>
>Joanne Fortune, Ph.D.
>Ithaca, New York
>
>Geula Gibori, Ph.D.
>Chicago, Illinois
>
>Julia Lobotsky, M.S.
>Bethesda, Maryland
>
>Richard Stouffer, Ph.D.
>Beaverton, Oregon
>
>Jerome Strauss III, M.D., Ph.D.
>Philadelphia, Pennsylvania

**Organizing Secretary**

>Bruce K. Burnett, Ph.D.
>Serono Symposia, USA
>100 Longwater Circle
>Norwell, Massachusetts

# Preface

The biennial Ovarian Workshops were created to provide a forum for scientists investigating the development and function of the ovary. These workshops bring together representatives of many disciplines in order to define important problems in ovarian physiology. The Ninth Ovarian Workshop was held at the University of North Carolina–Chapel Hill's Friday Continuing Education Center in Chapel Hill, North Carolina, as a satellite to the 1992 meeting of the Society for the Study of Reproduction. The 1992 workshop focused on the interaction between the cells of the ovary, from genes to physiology. Presentation sessions covered inhibin and activin, apoptosis, oocyte and early embryo development, gonadotropin receptor structure, follicle development and ovulation, and ovarian regulatory peptides. The present volume covers the talks given at the meeting, but does not include a record of the interesting discussion workshops on atresia and apoptosis, oocyte and early embryonic development, and corpus luteum and steroidogenesis. In addition, 97 posters and 6 Young Investigator slide presentations are not incorporated here.

Due to the introduction of molecular and cellular biology approaches, our understanding of ovarian physiology has reached a new level during the last few years. The present volume attempts to provide a new perspective on the ovary from molecular and cellular to whole-organ levels, from nonmammalian and rodent to human levels, and from paracrine, neuroendocrine, and endocrine levels as well.

The success of the Ovarian Workshop depends on the efforts of many individuals. We thank the other members of the Board of Directors (Drs. Eli Adashi, Jennifer Dorrington, John Eppig, Joanne Fortune, Geula Gibori, Julia Lobotsky, Richard Stouffer, and Jerome Strauss) for their work in organizing the program, choosing the speakers for each of the sessions, and chairing the various workshops. We also thank Serono Symposia, USA for both their continuing sponsorship of the Ovarian Workshop and their organization of the many details involved with this meeting; their support and involvement are important to the success of the Workshop. Most importantly, we thank the outstanding speakers for their talks and their timely contributions to this volume.

AARON J.W. HSUEH
DAVID W. SCHOMBERG

# Contents

Preface ............................................................. vii
Contributors ........................................................ xi

1. Apoptosis: Signal Transduction and Modes of Activation .... 1
   LU-ANN M. CARON-LESLIE AND JOHN A. CIDLOWSKI

### Part I.  Oocyte and Cell Cycle

2. Role of c-*kit* and Its Ligand in Oocyte Growth ............. 25
   ROSEMARY F. BACHVAROVA, KATIA MANOVA, ALAN I. PACKER,
   ERIC J. HUANG, AND PETER BESMER

3. Proteoglycan and Hyaluronic Acid Synthesis by Granulosa
   Cells: Regulation by an Oocyte Factor and Gonadotropins .. 38
   ANTONIETTA SALUSTRI, MASAKI YANAGISHITA, ANTONELLA
   CAMAIONI, EVELINA TIRONE, AND VINCENT C. HASCALL

4. Developmental Genetics of the Zona Pellucida ............ 49
   JURRIEN DEAN

5. Toward an Understanding of the Eukaryotic Cell Cycle:
   A Biochemical Approach ............................... 60
   HELEN PIWNICA-WORMS, SUE ATHERTON-FESSLER,
   MARGARET S. LEE, SCOTT OGG, AND LAURA L. PARKER

6. Hormonal Control of Cell-Cycle Checkpoints in Mammalian
   Oocytes ............................................... 79
   DAVID F. ALBERTINI, ANN E. ALLWORTH, AND
   SUSAN M. MESSINGER

### Part II.  Gonadotropin Receptor and Control Mechanisms

7. Structure and Regulation of the LH Receptor Gene and
   Its Transcripts ........................................ 89
   TAE H. JI, YONG BUM KOO, AND INHAE JI

8. Regulation of Expression of the FSH Receptor .............. 100
   MICHAEL D. GRISWOLD AND LESLIE L. HECKERT

9. Mouse Ovarian Prolactin Receptors ...................... 110
   DIANA L. CLARKE, KATHLEEN H. YOUNG, AND
   DANIEL I.H. LINZER

10. Molecular Regulation of Genes Involved in Ovulation and
    Luteinization .......................................... 125
    JOANNE S. RICHARDS, JEAN SIROIS, USHA NATRAJ, JACQUELINE
    K. MORRIS, SUSAN L. FITZPATRICK, AND JEFFREY W. CLEMENS

11. Dynamics of Human Follicle Development ................ 134
    BART C.J.M. FAUSER, THIERRY D. PACHE, AND DICK C. SCHOOT

## Part III. Intraovarian Regulatory Systems

12. Structural and Functional Studies of Insulin-Like Growth
    Factor Binding Proteins in the Ovary .................... 151
    N.C. LING, X.-J. LIU, M. MALKOWSKI, Y.-L. GUO,
    G.F. ERICKSON, AND S. SHIMASAKI

13. Luteotropic and Luteolytic Effects of Peptides in the Porcine
    and Human Corpus Luteum ............................ 167
    WOLFGANG WUTTKE, HUBERTUS JARRY, LUTZ PITZEL,
    EVA DIETRICH, AND SABINE SPIESS

14. A Role for Neurotrophic Factors in Ovarian Development ... 181
    SERGIO R. OJEDA, GREGORY A. DISSEN, SASHA MALAMED,
    AND ANNE N. HIRSHFIELD

Author Index ............................................. 203
Subject Index ............................................ 205

# Contributors

DAVID F. ALBERTINI, Tufts University School of Medicine, Boston, Massachusetts, USA.

ANN E. ALLWORTH, Tufts University School of Medicine, Boston, Massachusetts, USA.

SUE ATHERTON-FESSLER, Department of Physiology, Tufts University School of Medicine, Boston, Massachusetts, USA.

ROSEMARY F. BACHVAROVA, Department of Cell Biology and Anatomy, Cornell University Medical College, New York, New York, USA.

PETER BESMER, Molecular Biology Program, Sloan Kettering Institute, and Cornell University Graduate School of Medical Sciences, New York, New York, USA.

ANTONELLA CAMAIONI, Dipartimento di Sanitá Pubblica e Biologia Cellulare, 2nd University of Rome, Rome, Italy.

LU-ANN M. CARON-LESLIE, Department of Physiology, University of North Carolina, Chapel Hill, North Carolina, USA.

JOHN A. CIDLOWSKI, Lineberger Comprehensive Cancer Center Cell Biology Program and Department of Physiology, University of North Carolina, Chapel Hill, North Carolina, USA.

DIANA L. CLARKE, Departments of Biochemistry, Molecular Biology, and Cell Biology, Northwestern University, Evanston, Illinois, USA.

JEFFREY W. CLEMENS, Department of Cell Biology, Baylor College of Medicine, Houston, Texas, USA.

JURRIEN DEAN, Chief, Mammalian Developmental Biology Section, Laboratory of Cellular and Developmental Biology, NIDDK, National Institutes of Health, Bethesda, Maryland, USA.

EVA DIETRICH, Institute of Animal Husbandry and Genetics, University of Göttingen, Göttingen, Germany.

GREGORY A. DISSEN, Division of Neuroscience, Oregon Regional Primate Research Center, Beaverton, Oregon, USA.

GREGORY F. ERICKSON, Department of Reproductive Medicine, University of California–San Diego, La Jolla, California, USA.

BART C.J.M. FAUSER, Section of Reproductive Endocrinology and Fertility, Department of Obstetrics and Gynecology, Dijkzigt Academic Hospital and Erasmus University, Rotterdam, The Netherlands.

SUSAN L. FITZPATRICK, Department of Cell Biology, Baylor College of Medicine, Houston, Texas, USA.

MICHAEL D. GRISWOLD, Department of Biochemistry and Biophysics, Washington State University, Pullman, Washington, USA.

YILI GUO, Department of Molecular Endocrinology, The Whittier Institute for Diabetes and Endocrinology, La Jolla, California, USA.

VINCENT C. HASCALL, Bone Research Branch, National Institute of Dental Research, National Institutes of Health, Bethesda, Maryland, USA.

LESLIE L. HECKERT, Department of Biochemistry and Biophysics, Washington State University, Pullman, Washington, USA.

ANNE N. HIRSHFIELD, Department of Anatomy, University of Maryland, Baltimore, Maryland, USA.

ERIC J. HUANG, Molecular Biology Program, Sloan Kettering Institute, Cornell University Graduate School of Medical Sciences, New York, New York, USA.

HUBERTUS JARRY, Clinical and Experimental Endocrinology, Department of Obstetrics and Gynecology, University of Göttingen, Göttingen, Germany.

INHAE JI, Department of Molecular Biology, University of Wyoming, Laramie, Wyoming, USA.

TAE H. JI, Department of Molecular Biology, University of Wyoming, Laramie, Wyoming, USA.

YONG BUM KOO, Department of Molecular Biology, University of Wyoming, Laramie, Wyoming, USA.

MARGARET S. LEE, Department of Physiology, Tufts University School of Medicine, Boston, Massachusetts, USA.

NICHOLAS C. LING, Department of Molecular Endocrinology, The Whittier Institute for Diabetes and Endocrinology, La Jolla, California, USA.

DANIEL I.H. LINZER, Departments of Biochemistry, Molecular Biology, and Cell Biology, Northwestern University, Evanston, Illinois, USA.

XIN-JUN LIU, Department of Molecular Endocrinology, The Whittier Institute for Diabetes and Endocrinology, La Jolla, California, USA.

SASHA MALAMED, Department of Neuroscience and Cell Biology, University of Medicine and Dentistry of New Jersey—Robert Wood Johnson Medical School, Piscataway, New Jersey, USA.

MARCIA MALKOWSKI, Department of Molecular Endocrinology, The Whittier Institute for Diabetes and Endocrinology, La Jolla, California, USA.

KATIA MANOVA, Program in Molecular Biology, Sloan Kettering Institute, and Department of Cell Biology and Anatomy, Cornell University Medical College, New York, New York, USA.

SUSAN M. MESSINGER, Tufts University School of Medicine, Boston, Massachusetts, USA.

JACQUELINE K. MORRIS, Department of Cell Biology, Baylor College of Medicine, Houston, Texas, USA.

USHA NATRAJ, Department of Cell Biology, Baylor College of Medicine, Houston, Texas, USA, and Institute for Research in Reproduction, Parel, Bombay, India.

SCOTT OGG, Department of Physiology, Tufts University School of Medicine, Boston, Massachusetts, USA.

SERGIO R. OJEDA, Division of Neuroscience, Oregon Regional Primate Research Center, Beaverton, Oregon, USA.

THIERRY D. PACHE, Section of Reproductive Endocrinology and Fertility, Department of Obstetrics and Gynecology, Dijkzigt Academic Hospital and Erasmus University, Rotterdam, The Netherlands.

ALAN I. PACKER, Department of Cell Biology and Anatomy, Cornell University Graduate School of Medical Sciences, New York, New York, USA.

LAURA L. PARKER, Department of Physiology, Tufts University School of Medicine, Boston, Massachusetts, USA.

LUTZ PITZEL, Clinical and Experimental Endocrinology, Department of Obstetrics and Gynecology, University of Göttingen, Göttingen, Germany.

HELEN PIWNICA-WORMS, Department of Physiology, Tufts University School of Medicine, Boston, Massachusetts, USA.

JOANNE S. RICHARDS, Department of Cell Biology, Baylor College of Medicine, Houston, Texas, USA.

ANTONIETTA SALUSTRI, Dipartimento di Sanitá Pubblica e Biologia Cellulare, 2nd University of Rome, Rome, Italy.

DICK C. SCHOOT, Section of Reproductive Endocrinology and Fertility, Department of Obstetrics and Gynecology, Dijkzigt Academic Hospital and Erasmus University, Rotterdam, The Netherlands.

SHUNICHI SHIMASAKI, Department of Molecular Endocrinology, The Whittier Institute for Diabetes and Endocrinology, La Jolla, California, USA.

JEAN SIROIS, Department of Cell Biology, Baylor College of Medicine, Houston, Texas, USA.

SABINE SPIESS, Clinical and Experimental Endocrinology, Department of Obstetrics and Gynecology, University of Göttingen, Göttingen, Germany.

EVELINA TIRONE, Dipartimento di Sanitá Pubblica e Biologia Cellulare, 2nd University of Rome, Rome, Italy.

WOLFGANG WUTTKE, Clinical and Experimental Endocrinology, Department of Obstetrics and Gynecology, University of Göttingen, Göttingen, Germany.

MASAKI YANAGISHITA, Bone Research Branch, National Institute of Dental Research, National Institutes of Health, Bethesda, Maryland, USA.

KATHLEEN H. YOUNG, Departments of Biochemistry, Molecular Biology, and Cell Biology, Northwestern University, Evanston, Illinois, USA.

# 1

# Apoptosis: Signal Transduction and Modes of Activation

Lu-Ann M. Caron-Leslie and John A. Cidlowski

The ability to maintain cellular populations is essential to the proper homeostatic function of organisms. This is accomplished through the finely orchestrated balance of cellular proliferation, differentiation, and death. Beginning early in development, certain cells within a population are chosen to proliferate and differentiate while neighboring cells are selectively deleted from that tissue. An excellent example of this coordinated selection of cellular populations is the embryonic limb bud. The limb bud first forms as a mass of cells with no discernible specialization; however, as differentiation occurs and digits are formed, the cells between the digits die, allowing the paw, or hand, to take shape.

The programming of certain cells to die while neighboring cells live is a genetically conserved process called *programmed cell death*, or *apoptosis*, and is found in many organisms ranging from nematodes to humans. In this chapter, we present an overview of what is currently known about the process of programmed cell death, or apoptosis, with an emphasis on the immune system where the most mechanistic information is available.

## Occurrence in Physiology and Pathology

Programmed cell death is prevalent in a multitude of diverse animal systems. For example, the nematode *C. elegans* has a well-defined pattern of cellular deletion during development (1). Apoptosis is also responsible for the loss of tissues during metamorphosis in amphibians and insects (2, 3). In higher organisms, programmed cell death is an integral part of normal embryonic development (4, 5). Apoptosis is also responsible for cell death in hormone-dependent tissues, such as breast (6), adrenal (7), prostate (8, 9), endometrium (10), and ovary (11–13).

Apoptosis is particularly prevalent in the immune system. In the thymus and in cell lines derived from thymocytes, programmed cell death results from the addition of glucocorticoid hormones (14–20). Many leukemias also exhibit apoptosis in response to glucocorticoid treatment (17, 21). Lymphoid tissues that are dependent on growth factors, such as IL-2-dependent lymphocytes (22) and IL-3-dependent hemopoietic precursors (23), often exhibit programmed cell death upon growth factor withdrawal. Autoreactive T cell clones within the thymus are deleted by programmed cell death (24), as are B cells that do not encounter the appropriate antigen (25). In addition, *natural killer* (NK) cells and *cytotoxic T lymphocytes* (CTL) cause death to their target cells through programmed cell death (26–28). Apoptosis is also responsible for the clearance of aged neutrophils following inflammation (29).

In addition to the previous physiological examples of apoptosis, there are also instances of apoptosis in pathology. Programmed cell death occurs in tumors (30–32) and plays an important role in the rate of tumor growth. What may appear to be a tumor with a high mitotic rate may actually be a tumor with a decreased proportion of apoptotic cells. B and T leukemic cells will undergo programmed cell death following treatment with monoclonal antibodies against APO-1, a specific surface epitope (33, 34). Cell death caused by chemotherapeutic agents (35, 36), toxin exposure (37–41), ionizing radiation (42–46), and, in the appropriate target cells, tumor necrosis factor (48) also occurs through apoptosis.

As illustrated above, programmed cell death can be triggered by a variety of signals. Indeed, the initiating signals for apoptosis are as diverse as the cell types in which apoptosis occurs. For example, steroid hormone-associated apoptosis is mediated through steroid hormone receptors that act by altering gene expression, whereas cell-surface receptors, such as the T cell receptor, transduce the apoptotic signal in the deletion of autoreactive thymocytes. In addition, the apoptotic stimulus may not be external; rather, it may be part of the genetic program that is expressed upon reaching a certain stage of differentiation, as in aged neutrophils (29). Although the signals mediating apoptosis are cell type specific, the initial stimulus does not seem to affect the final outcome; the cell undergoes characteristic morphological and biochemical events and dies without activating an immune response.

## Morphological Changes Associated with Apoptosis

When considering cell death, it is common to imagine necrotic death that results from a toxic injury. In this instance, the cell loses its ability to produce and use ATP. The transporters at the cellular membrane that maintain the intracellular ionic environment are unable to function, resulting in an increase in intracellular volume, and the cell appears to swell (48). Intracellular organelles also lose membrane integrity and similarly increase in volume. Finally, the cellular membrane breaks apart, and cellular contents are released into the extracellular spaces. In complex organisms such as humans, this is a potentially disastrous situation since the release of intracellular material would trigger an immunological response, resulting in inflammation and further tissue injury.

In all of the tissues where programmed cell death or apoptosis occurs, a common morphology that is easily distinguished from necrosis is observed. This characteristic morphology occurs in three recognizable stages (49–53). In the first stage, there is a loss of cell volume, in contrast to the increase in cell volume observed during necrosis. This is due, in part, to dilation of the endoplasmic reticulum, resulting in the formation of vesicles that fuse to the plasma membrane and extrude vesicular contents (54). The apoptotic cell then shrinks away from surrounding cells and loses microvilli, resulting in a smooth cellular contour with a convoluted outline. Although the organelles remain essentially intact, they become compacted within the cell. The nucleus, however, is altered considerably. The nucleoli disintegrate, and the chromatin condenses, forming "beads" along the nuclear envelope.

In the second stage of apoptosis, blebs consisting of organelles within intact membrane are formed along the outer surface of the cell. Upon time-lapse photography the cell actually seems to boil (55) as the blebs appear upon the cell surface. These blebs, known as *apoptotic bodies*, are usually phagocytosed by surrounding cells and macrophages (56). The disposal of the dying cells by surrounding cells and macrophages insures that intracellular contents are not released and, thus, will not result in an inflammatory response.

In the third stage of apoptosis, the apoptotic bodies that are not phagocytosed lose membrane integrity and rupture (57), a process termed *secondary necrosis*. Only at this point do they become permeable to such vital dyes as trypan blue. In many cell culture systems used to study programmed cell death, the third stage of the apoptotic process is often not fulfilled since there are no surrounding cells capable of phagocytosis.

# Biochemical Events Associated with Apoptosis

Although there are common morphological changes in all cells dying through apoptosis, many of the biochemical initiators are cell type specific because of the need for selectivity. There are, however, two common biochemical events associated with almost all instances of apoptosis. The first common biochemical characteristic is the degradation of DNA into fragments consisting of multiples of 180–200 bp. This pattern of DNA degradation has become the biochemical hallmark of apoptosis and has been used by many investigators to determine if cell death is occurring through apoptotic mechanisms.

The second common characteristic of apoptosis is phagocytosis of apoptotic cells, which depends on biochemical alterations in the cell membrane that permit subsequent recognition by phagocytic cells. There are obviously many other biochemical events that are associated with apoptosis, including the cell type-specific signaling pathways of apoptotic triggers. As additional research is performed, we will undoubtedly learn which intracellular mechanisms are common to all cells undergoing apoptosis, as well as those that are cell type specific. Given the complex phenotypes of cells that can undergo apoptosis, there is no reason to believe that all cells will die in precisely the same way.

## Common Biochemical Events Associated with Apoptosis

### DNA Degradation

*Internucleosomal DNA degradation*—that is, cleavage of chromatin into fragments of multiples of 180–200 bp—has been detected in most systems where the apoptotic morphology has been described. These include glucocorticoid-treated thymocytes and thymocyte cell lines (14–20, 58), thymocytes treated with antibodies against the T cell receptor (59), thymocytes treated with calcium ionophores (60, 61), uterine epithelium following ovariectomy (10), and prostate following castration (62). Figure 1.1 shows an example of internucleosomal DNA degradation in glucocorticoid-treated S49 mouse lymphoma cells and illustrates that the glucocorticoid-mediated internucleosomal DNA degradation is inhibited by the glucocorticoid receptor antagonist RU 486. This form of DNA degradation is not seen in instances of necrotic cell death (63). The occurrence of internucleosomal DNA degradation has been accepted as the biochemical hallmark of apoptosis and has been used by many investigators to determine if the cell death that they are observing is due to apoptotic mechanisms.

Several pieces of evidence suggest that DNA degradation is the irreversible step in the apoptotic cascade that is necessary for death to occur. DNA degradation occurs prior to cell death (14, 16) and, in some systems, transcription and translation are necessary for both DNA degradation and cell death (64). In addition, *aurintricarboxylic acid* (ATA), a general nuclease inhibitor, and zinc inhibit not only DNA degradation but cell death as well (58, 64). These compounds also inhibit internucleosomal cleavage activity in protein extracts from apoptotic thymocyte nuclei in an assay where nuclei from apoptotic deficient cells are used as a substrate for nucleases (Schwartzman, Cidlowski, unpublished observations). Interestingly, calcium and magnesium, which are essential for cell death (15, 60), are also required for the internucleosomal cleavage

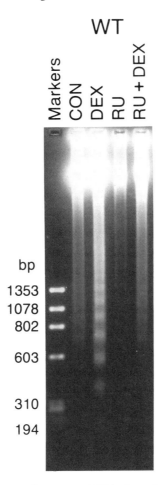

FIGURE 1.1. Effect of dexamethasone on DNA degradation in S49 cells. S49 cells were treated with vehicle, dexamethasone (DEX, 0.1 μM), the glucocorticoid antagonist RU 486 (RU, 1.0 μM), or RU plus DEX (1.0 μM and 0.1 μM, respectively) for 18 h. DNA was isolated from live cells as previously described in reference 19 and electrophoresed on 1.8% agarose gels (15 μg/lane). The gels were stained with ethidium bromide (0.5 μg/mL) and photographed. The results shown are representative of 4 experiments. Reprinted with permission from Caron-Leslie and Cidlowski (18), © by The Endocrine Society, 1991.

activity of the thymocyte nuclease (Schwartzman, Cidlowski, unpublished observations).

Finally, it is of interest that when nuclei from untreated thymocytes are incubated with micrococcal nuclease (a bacterial nuclease that has internucleosomal cleavage activity) and protease inhibitors, not only is the DNA cleaved internucleosomally, but the nuclei exhibit the morphological changes characteristic of apoptosis (65). Together, these findings pro-

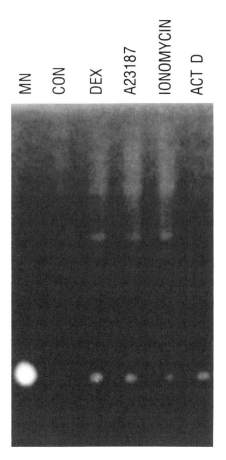

FIGURE 1.2. Nuclease activity in nuclear extracts of apoptotic S49 cells. S49 cells were treated with vehicle, dexamethasone (DEX, 0.1 µM), A23187 (250 nM), ionomycin (2.5 µM), or actinomycin D (56 nM) for 18 h, harvested, and 0.3 M NaCl nuclear extracts prepared as described in reference 19. Nuclear extracts (2.5 µg) were analyzed for nuclease activity following electrophoresis through 15% polyacrylamide gels (with 750,000-cpm, $^{32}$P-labeled calf thymus DNA incorporated within the gel matrix) by soaking the gel to remove the SDS and adding calcium and magnesium for 24 h at 37°C to activate nucleases. (See reference 19 for detailed methods.) The gel was then dired down, and an autoradiograph was prepared by exposing the gel to X-ray film for 6 h at −70°C. The clear areas on the autoradiograph reflect the locations of nucleases that have degraded the radiolabeled DNA within the gel matrix. Micrococcal nuclease, an 18-kd nuclease, was used as a positive control (MN, 0.5 µg). The results shown are representative of at least 4 experiments.

vide strong evidence that DNA degradation is a precipitating event in apoptosis. Once the nuclease responsible for the internucleosomal cleavage activity in apoptotic cells is purified and cloned, this hypothesis can be tested.

One candidate for the apoptotic nuclease (NUC18) has recently been purified from glucocorticoid-treated rat thymocytes (66). Figure 1.2 shows that this 18-kd nuclease is also found in nuclear extracts of S49 mouse lymphoma cells undergoing apoptosis in response to treatment with a variety of compounds, including glucocorticoids, either of two calcium ionophores—A23187 or ionomycin—or actinomycin D. This nuclease also results from the treatment of S49 cells with inhibitors of DNA or protein synthesis (Caron-Leslie, Cidlowski, unpublished observations). Further studies are necessary, however, to determine if this is the nuclease responsible for the internucleosomal degradation that is associated with apoptotic death.

Finally, what mechanisms are responsible for expression of the nuclease activity? One possibility is that the nuclease is synthesized de novo. Evidence supporting this notion includes the finding that transcription and translation are necessary for DNA degradation and apoptosis in some systems (60). Other systems have been found, however, where intact transcription and translation are not necessary for apoptosis to occur (67, 68), and inhibition of transcription and translation can sometimes cause apoptosis (69–72; Caron-Leslie, Cidlowski, unpublished observations). Another finding that refutes the de novo synthesis hypothesis is that internucleosomal DNA degradation is observed when rat thymocyte nuclei are incubated with calcium and magnesium, a phenomenon termed *autodigestion* (15). For this to occur, the nuclease would have to be present within the nuclei prior to glucocorticoid treatment.

Other possible modes of nuclease activity expression are activation of an inactive precursor, disinhibition of a repressed nuclease, or, perhaps, translocation of an active nuclease from the cytoplasm to the nucleus. It is possible that a combination of mechanisms is responsible for the expression of nuclease activity and that there is a cell type-specific component involved. Perhaps in some cell types a protein must be synthesized that relieves the inhibition of the nuclease or must work in concert with increased calcium concentrations to allow the expression of an active nuclease, whereas in other cell types increased calcium concentrations alone can activate the nuclease. Many questions remain to be answered concerning this aspect of apoptotic biochemistry. Since this remains a very active and growing field of research, some of these questions will surely be answered in the near future.

Phagocyte Recognition

In vivo, apoptotic cells are phagocytosed by macrophages and surrounding cells. It would seem that some membrane component must be altered to allow phagocytic cells to recognize these apoptotic cells. Phagocytosis of rodent thymocytes is inhibited by N-acetylglucosamine (73), while phagocytosis of aging neutrophils is inhibited by galactosamine, mannosamine, and glucosamine (74). These data suggest that a lectin-like recognition process is responsible. Phagocytosis is also inhibited by fibronectin, vitronectin, monoclonal antibodies against the vitronectin receptor, and the RGDS tetrapeptide that serves as the recognition sequence for the vitronectin receptor (75). Obviously, some component of the apoptotic cell membrane must be interacting with preexisting receptors on macrophages or similar phagocytic cells. The membrane components on the apoptotic cell remain unidentified; however, they may be carried to the cell surface through the fusion of vesicles originating from the endoplasmic reticulum. Recently, an enzymatic mechanism for the expression of specific phospholipids on the outer membrane that are normally found on the inner membrane has also been proposed (76). Since there appears to be cooperativity between different mechanisms (77), it is possible that more than one mechanism may be responsible for the recognition of apoptotic cells by its neighbors and macrophages.

## Cell Type-Specific Signaling Pathways in Apoptosis

### Calcium

Glucocorticoid-induced lymphocytolysis was the model of apoptosis used to determine if calcium was important to the apoptotic process. In the early 1980s, it was found that glucocorticoid-induced apoptosis was inhibited when thymocytes were treated in vitro in calcium-free media. In addition, the calcium ionophore A23187 could stimulate internucleosomal DNA degradation in thymocytes (60), and A23187 or another calcium ionophore, ionomycin, similarly caused internucleosomal DNA degradation in both glucocorticoid-responsive and glucocorticoid-resistant S49 mouse lymphoma cells (18). Internucleosomal DNA degradation was found in thymocyte nuclei that were incubated with calcium and magnesium (15).

It was also found that apoptotic cells exhibited an increase in $[Ca^{++}]_i$, although these studies did not determine if the increase had occurred prior to cell death (78, 79). More recent studies have confirmed that a sustained increase in $[Ca^{++}]_i$ is an early event following the glucocorticoid treatment of thymocytes in vitro (61). The elevation in intracellular calcium is not observed in calcium-free media and is suppressed by such calcium-quenching compounds as quin-2, as well as by inhibitors of protein synthesis (80). These findings suggest that the increase in $[Ca^{++}]_i$ following glucocorticoid treatment results from the influx of calcium from extracellular media and may involve de novo synthesis of a calcium channel or an activator of a preexisting calcium channel.

Gliotoxin-induced apoptosis in macrophages has been associated with the formation of *inositol triphosphate* ($IP_3$) (40), a compound known to mobilize intracellular calcium stores, although this report did not include intracellular calcium measurements. An $IP_3$-mediated increase in $[Ca^{++}]_i$ has been associated with apoptosis in thymocytes treated with monoclonal antibodies against the T cell receptor and CD3 surface antigen (59, 81).

Increased intracellular calcium concentrations are not always associated with cell death, however. The role of calcium as a second messenger in lymphocytes is complicated by the different responses that these cells have to calcium at different stages of maturation. For example, in mature lymphocytes, concomitant treatment with compounds that increase $[Ca^{++}]_i$ and compounds that activate protein kinase C can result in activation of the lymphocyte and mitosis rather than apoptosis. In contrast, the immature thymocyte responds to the increase in intracellular calcium through apoptosis, suggesting that the differentiation state of the cell is important to the control of intracellular pathways.

Other immune responses that involve apoptosis also involve calcium. For example, upon CTL activation, lytic granules are released that attack the target cell (82). A component of the lytic granule is perforin, a pore-forming molecule that renders the target cell permeable to ions. Similarly, apoptosis in target cells attacked by NK cells involves an increase in intracellular calcium concentration (83).

Calcium has also been implicated in apoptosis in three other systems: the prostate, the liver, and neurons. In the rat prostate, the calcium ionophore A23187 can mimic withdrawal of testosterone in the induction of apoptosis (9). Furthermore, nifedipine, a calcium channel blocker, inhibited cell death resulting from the removal of testosterone. Programmed cell death in hepatocytes following *2,3,7,8-tetrachlorodibenzo-p-dioxin* (TCDD) exposure also involves a sustained increase in $[Ca^{++}]_i$ (41) derived from the influx of calcium from extracellular pools. In addition, a calmodulin-dependent calcium transporter that is stimulated by ATP and mediates calcium uptake by the nucleus (84) has been identified in hepatocytes, although the role of this transporter in apoptosis has not been fully elucidated. In contrast to these reports, however, calcium has a protective effect on programmed cell death in sympathetic neurons deprived of nerve growth factor (85). Finally, increased intracellular calcium concentrations are not always associated with apoptosis or mitosis. Although calcium ionophore treatment of HeLa cells causes cell death, cellular DNA is not degraded in the internucleosomal pattern characteristic of apoptosis, indicating that cell death is most probably due to necrosis rather than apoptosis (18).

How is calcium working to activate apoptosis? An increase in $[Ca^{++}]_i$ has been implicated in apoptotic effects on the cell membrane and in DNA degradation. In the cell membrane, increased intracellular calcium concentrations can lead to the dissociation of actin microfilaments from alpha actinin, an intermediate in the association of microfilaments with actin binding proteins, thereby disrupting the plasma membrane anchor. In addition, certain cytoskeletal changes that occur during apoptosis are mediated through the calcium-dependent activation of transglutaminase (86). Calcium-dependent phospholipases (87–89) and neutral proteases (90, 91) may also be involved in these membrane alterations. Intracellular calcium may be working through the activation of calcium-calmodulin-dependent enzymes. In thymocytes, inhibitors of calmodulin inhibit glucocorticoid-mediated DNA degradation, but have no effect on the increase in $[Ca^{++}]_i$ (58). In addition, glucocorticoids increase the level of calmodulin mRNA (92). These findings suggest that calcium-calmodulin-dependent enzymes are integral to the apoptotic mechanisms induced by glucocorticoids.

Finally, as we have discussed in the previous section, calcium is also involved in the DNA degradation observed in apoptosis. Not only is calcium necessary to activate the nuclease itself (15, 58, 60), but calcium may also act as a second messenger (58). Additional research is necessary to determine if calcium plays a role in many of the other cell types in which apopotic cell death occurs.

Protein Kinase C

Intracellular signaling pathways that involve *protein kinase C* (PKC) have also been implicated in the regulation of apoptosis. Phorbol esters that activate PKC protect thymocytes from the DNA degradation and cell death resulting from anti-T cell receptor antibodies and calcium ionophores (59, 93). Interleukin-1, a physiological activator of PKC, had a similar effect on anti-T cell receptor antibody-induced apoptosis, but did not prevent the increase in intracellular calcium concentration (94). Phorbol esters also protected leukemic cells from apoptosis caused by topoisomerase II-reactive chemotherapeutic agents (95) and cytochalasin B-induced apoptosis in T lymphocytes (96). Cytochalasin B acts through the inhibition of actin filament polymerization and, in this example, PKC appears to be acting by enhancing polymerization of actin filaments (97, 98).

The mechanism of action of PKC in the previous examples remains undetermined. It is obvious, however, that PKC plays a part in the apoptotic process, and regulation of PKC may be involved in the differential apoptotic regulation of immature thymocytes and mature lymphocytes. There is, however, some controversy about the effect of PKC in apoptosis when H-7, a PKC inhibitor, has been studied. H-7 was found to inhibit glucocorticoid- and A23187-induced apoptosis in thymocytes (99, 100), suggesting that PKC is essential for glucocorticoid and A23187 action. It is possible, however, that H-7 inhibits other kinases in addition to PKC and that they are responsible for the observed effect. As more information accumulates concerning the role of PKC in apoptosis and the PKC substrates relevant to the apoptotic process, it will be possible to determine what is responsible for these conflicting reports. It is not known if PKC plays a role in apoptosis in nonlymphoid cells.

Cyclic AMP

Another level of apoptotic regulation is mediated through cAMP-dependent protein kinases. Cyclic AMP has been found to mediate cell death exhibiting the characteristic apoptotic morphology in embryonic palatal shelf tissue (101), cell culture systems, and carcinogen-induced animal tumors (102). Recently, investigators have found that agents that increase intracellular cAMP levels (forskolin, *prostaglandin* $E_2$ [$PGE_2$]; cholera toxin, and adenosine) and cAMP analogs cause cell death that is associated with internucleosomal DNA degradation in leukemic cell lines (103), mouse thymocytes, and T lymphocytes (104, 105). There is controversy concerning whether the effect of cAMP involves calcium, however. McConkey et al. (105) detected no increase in intracellular calcium concentration following treatment of mouse thymocytes with $PGE_2$, whereas Kelley et al. (106) detected a rise in intracellular calcium concentration concomitant with the increase in cAMP following treatment of the Jurkat T lymphocyte cell line with $PGE_2$, forskolin, and cAMP analogs. The difference in these two reports could be due to an alteration in intracellular signaling that occurs when thymocytes differentiate to mature lymphocytes or, perhaps, to a phenotypic alteration resulting from the acclimation of the lymphocytes to cell culture conditions.

Cyclic AMP also modulates the effect of other apoptotic activators. Cyclic AMP has been found to potentiate glucocorticoid effects by increasing the number of glucocorticoid receptors (107). Conversely, glucocorticoids can potentiate the effect of cAMP by inhibiting the phosphodiesterase that is responsible for converting cAMP to AMP (108). Together, these possibilities illustrate the potential for multilevel regulation of apoptosis within a cell and how cross talk between different intracellular signaling pathways can influence the apoptotic mechanism in various tissues. In addition, it is obvious that not all cell types respond to increased cAMP levels through apoptotic mechanisms. Elucidating how these signaling pathways influence each other will be necessary to understand fully the regulation of apoptosis.

Protein Synthesis and Gene Expression

One of the first components of the apoptotic mechanism to be described was inhibition of glucocorticoid-induced thymocytolysis by cycloheximide, suggesting that de novo protein synthesis was essential to apoptosis (15, 20, 60). This was not very surprising since glucocorticoids are known to act through the regulation of gene expression. It was subsequently reported, however, that apoptosis was dependent on protein synthesis in other systems as well, including IL-2-deprived T cell lines and T lymphoblasts (109), irradiated thymocytes (110), activation-induced death of T cell hybridomas (111, 112), antibodies against CD3 in thymocytes (113), thymocytes treated with chemotherapeutic agents (114), and calcium ionophores (60). From these reports and many others, it was expected that de novo protein synthesis would be a requirement in all systems examined.

Recently, however, several exceptions to this assumption have been reported. Cycloheximide did not inhibit apoptosis mediated by valinomycin (115), cytotoxic T lymphocytes (116), gliotoxin-treated macrophages (40), primary leukemia cells (67), hyperthermia in thymocytes (117), and tumor cell lines (118). In addition, systems were found where cycloheximide was a potent inducer of apoptosis, including S49 mouse lymphoma cells (119 and Caron-Leslie, Cidlowski, unpublished observations), HL-60 cells (69) and other hemopoietic cell lines (71), concanavalin A-stimulated T blasts and macrophages (40), and B chronic lymphocytic leukemia cells (72). In addition, actinomycin D, a transcription inhibitor, similarly induced apoptosis in gastrointestinal crypts (120) and in S49 mouse lymphoma cells (Caron-Leslie, Cidlowski, unpublished observations). Obviously, the dependence on protein synthesis must be evaluated in each system where apoptosis occurs. This suggests that certain cell types have all the components of the apoptotic cascade resident within the cell but under the regulation of an inhibitor or activator, providing still another level of regulation.

Many examples of altered gene expression in different apoptotic systems have been reported; unfortunately, the function of regulated genes is not often known. Perhaps the most thoroughly studied is *Caenorhabditis elegans*. The fate of nearly all cells in this organism is known, and mutants are available that exhibit inhibited cell death (121). Two genes have been identified (ced3 and ced4) that are capable of blocking cell death (1). In the tobacco hornworm, *Manduca sexta*, 4 genes have been identified that are expressed when cells commit to die (122). Genes induced during glucocorticoid- and cAMP-induced apoptosis in thymoma cell lines have also been studied, and 11 inducible genes have been isolated (123), but none has been directly linked to the activation of apoptosis.

Several other specific genes have been identified, although the significance of the modulated genes is not understood. In apoptotic neonatal rat liver, transglutaminase is activated (124). In glucocorticoid-treated lymphoma cell lines, the expression of c-*erb*A protooncogene is increased (125), while there is a decrease in the expression of c-*myc*, c-*myb*, and c-Ki-*ras* (126). Conversely, c-*myc* is up-regulated in apoptotic liver along with c-*fos* (127). In prostate, there is also an increase in c-*fos* and c-*myc*, as well as *hsp*70 and TGFβ (8, 128). *Testosterone-repressed prostate* *message 2* (TRPM2) is also found in apoptotic prostate, and its expression is maximal when the cell death rate is maximal (129, 130). The significance of TRPM2 to apoptosis is unclear, however, especially since it has been found in nonapoptotic tissues (131), including normal testis (132).

Recently, a gene has been found (BCL2) that appears to confer apoptotic resistance in myeloid cells and pro-B cells without inducing proliferation (133). The BCL2 protein localizes to the inner mitochondrial membrane (134) and is found in long-lived stem cells, neurons, glandular epithelia, lymphoid germinal centers, and the surviving cells of the thymic medulla (135). BCL2 does not inhibit apoptosis induced by the withdrawal of IL-2 or IL-6 (136), however. The function of BCL2 remains to be determined.

Steroid Hormone Regulation of Apoptosis

Steroid hormones can be either essential or detrimental to the viability of a variety of cell types. The addition of glucocorticoids causes apoptosis in thymocytes (14–16), whereas the removal of androgens and estrogens mediates apoptosis in prostate (8, 137, 138) and breast tissue (139), respectively. Similarly, a loss of progesterone induces apoptosis in uterine epithelium (10, 140), whereas an increase in progesterone levels may be involved in the apoptosis of ovarian granulosa cells observed during follicular atresia (12). In all cases that have been studied, the respective steroid antagonist reverses either the protective or apoptotic effect of the steroid hormone (16, 18–20, 140, 141), indicating that the steroids are acting through classical steroid hormone mechanisms involving a steroid hormone receptor. Following interaction with a steroid receptor, the steroid receptor is activated, and the receptor is then able to bind to specific DNA sequences. Specific interactions between the steroid receptor and DNA result in altered gene expression. In this way, the addition or removal of steroid hormones can also result in the increase or decrease in the level of specific proteins.

In the previous section we have seen that this has been observed in steroid-mediated apoptosis. Specifically, estrogen ablation-induced apoptosis in estrogen-dependent breast cancer cells and androgen ablation-induced apoptosis in prostate are associated with an increase in both TGFβ and TRPM2 (62, 138, 139). TGFβ is known to have antiproliferative effects and induces apoptosis in uterine epithelial cells (142), whereas the role of TRPM2 remains unclear. Glucocorticoid-mediated apoptosis in thymocytes may involve the synthesis of a novel calcium transporter (80). Calcium also seems to be involved in androgen ablation-induced apoptosis in prostate since a calcium channel blocker reversed the protective effects of testosterone (143). Exactly what genes are responsible for steroid-mediated apoptosis remains unclear. The function of specific proteins identified to date is mostly unknown, as discussed previously. Further research is necessary to determine exactly what mediates steroid-induced apoptosis.

## Conclusion

The ability to delete unwanted cells, unneeded cells, or cells whose presence may be detrimental to the proper function of the organism through apoptosis appears to be a genetically conserved phenomenon that is essential to homeostasis. Although the signals that trigger the apoptotic response are as varied as the tissues in which apoptosis has been observed, common mechanisms appear to be responsible for the actual death of the cell. We propose that the apoptotic mechanisms are resident within all cells, but under various forms of regulation. In this way, apoptotic cell death would be the default mechanism capable of protecting and maintaining the organism as a whole. Although research into apoptotic cell death has increased almost exponentially within the past five years, much more remains to be determined concerning the biochemical mechanisms involved in this type of cell death.

*Acknowledgment.* This work was supported by NIH Grant DK-32078.

## *References*

1. Ellis HM, Horvitz HR. Genetic control of programmed cell death in the nematode *C. elegans*. Cell 1986;44:817–29.
2. Kerr JFR, Harmon B, Searle J. An electron-microscope study of cell deletion in the anuran tadpole tail during spontaneous metamorphosis with special reference to apoptosis of striated muscle fibres. Cell Sci 1974;14:571–85.
3. Wadewitz AG, Lockshin RA. Programmed cell death: dying cells synthesize a coordinated, unique set of proteins in two different episodes of cell death. FEBS Lett 1988;241:19–23.
4. Hurle JM. Cell death in developing systems. Methods Achiev Exp Pathol 1988;13:55–86.
5. Clarke PGH. Developmental cell death: morphological diversity and multiple mechanisms. Anat Embryol (Berl) 1990;181:195–213.
6. Walker NI, Bennett RE, Kerr JFR. Cell death by apoptosis during involution of the lactating breast in mice and rats. Am J Anat 1989;185:19–32.
7. Wyllie AH, Kerr JFR, Macaskill IAM, Currie AR. Adrenocortical cell deletion: the role of ACTH. J Pathol 1973;111:85–94.
8. Kyprianou N, Isaacs JT. Activation of programmed cell death in the rat ventral prostate after castration. Endocrinology 1988;122:552–62.
9. Martikainen P, Isaacs J. Role of calcium in the programmed death of rat prostatic glandular cells. Prostate 1990;17:175–7.

10. Rotello RJ, Hocker MB, Gerschenson LE. Biochemical evidence for programmed cell death in rabbit uterine epithelium. Am J Pathol 1989; 134:491–5.
11. Zeleznik AJ, Ihrig LL, Bassett SG. Developmental expression of $Ca^{++}$/$Mg^{++}$-dependent endonuclease activity in rat granulosa and luteal cells. Endocrinology 1989;125:2218–20.
12. Hughes FM Jr, Gorospe WC. Biochemical identification of apoptosis (programmed cell death) in granulosa cells: evidence for a potential mechanism underlying follicular atresia. Endocrinology 1991;129:2415–22.
13. Tilly JL, Kowalski KI, Johnson AL, Hsueh AJW. Involvement of apoptosis in ovarian follicular atresia and postovulatory regression. Endocrinology 1991;129:2799–801.
14. Wyllie AH. Glucocorticoid-induced thymocyte apoptosis is associated with endogenous endonuclease activation. Nature 1980;284:555–6.
15. Cohen JJ, Duke RC. Glucocorticoid activation of a calcium-dependent endonuclease in thymocyte nuclei leads to cell death. J Immuol 1984; 132:38–42.
16. Compton MM, Cidlowski JA. Rapid in vivo effects of glucocorticoids on the integrity of rat lymphocyte genomic deoxyribonucleic acid. Endocrinology 1986;118:38–45.
17. Distelhorst CW. Glucocorticosteroids induce DNA fragmentation in human lymphoid leukemia cells. Blood 1988;72:1305–9.
18. Caron-Leslie LM, Cidlowski JA. Similar actions of glucocorticoids and calcium on the regulation of apoptosis in S49 cells. Mol Endocrinol 1991; 5:1169–79.
19. Compton MM, Cidlowski JA. Identification of a glucocorticoid-induced nuclease in thymocytes. A potential "lysis gene" product. J Biol Chem 1987;262:8288–92.
20. Compton MM, Haskill JS, Cidlowski JA. Analysis of glucocorticoid actions on rat thymocyte deoxyribonucleic acid by fluorescence-activated flow cytometry. Endocrinology 1988;122:2158–64.
21. McConkey DJ, Aguilar-Santelises M, Hartzell P, et al. Induction of DNA fragmentation in chronic B-lymphocytic leukemia cells. J Immunol 1991; 146:1072–6.
22. Nieto MA, Gonzalez A, Lopez-Rivas A, Diaz-Espada F, Gambon F. IL-2 protects against anti-CD3-induced cell death in human medullary thymocytes. J Immunol 1990;145:1364–8.
23. Williams GT, Smith CA, Spooncer E, Dexter TM, Taylor DR. Haemopoietic colony stimulating factors promote cell survival by suppressing apoptosis. Nature 1990;343:76–9.
24. Smith CA, Williams GT, Kingston R, Jenkinson EJ, Owen JJT. Antibodies to CD3/T-cell receptor complex induce death by apoptosis in immature T cells in thymic cultures. Nature 1989;337:181–4.
25. Hasbold J, Klaus GGB. Anti-immunoglobulin antibodies induce apoptosis in immature B cell lymphomas. Eur J Immunol 1990;20:1685–90.
26. Duke RC, Cohen JJ, Chervenak R. Differences in target cell DNA fragmentation induced by mouse cytotoxic T lymphocytes and natural killer cells. J Immunol 1986;137:1442–7.
27. Duvall E, Wyllie AH. Death and the cell. Immunol Today 1986;7:115–9.

28. Zychlinsky A, Zheng LM, Liu C-C, Young JD-E. Cytolytic lymphocytes induce both apoptosis and necrosis in target cells. J Immunol 1991;146: 393–400.
29. Savill JS, Henson PM, Haslett C. Phagocytosis of aged human neutrophils by macrophages is mediated by a novel "charge-sensitive" recognition mechanism. J Clin Invest 1989;84:1518–27.
30. Kerr JFR, Wyllie AH, Currie AR. Apoptosis: a basic biological phenomenon with wide-ranging implications in tissue kinetics. Br J Cancer 1972;26: 239–57.
31. Sarraf CE, Bowen ID. Kinetic studies on a murine sarcoma and an analysis of apoptosis. Br J Cancer 1986;54:989–98.
32. El-Labban NG, Osorio-Herrera E. Apoptotic bodies and abnormally dividing epithelial cells in squamous cell carcinoma. Histopathology 1986;10:921–31.
33. Trauth BC, Klas C, Peters AMJ, et al. Monoclonal antibody-mediated tumor regression by induction of apoptosis. Science 1989;245:301–4.
34. Debatin K-M, Goldmann CK, Bamford R, Waldmann TA, Krammer PH. Monoclonal-antibody-mediated apoptosis in adult T-cell leukaemia. Lancet 1990;335:497–500.
35. Barry MA, Behnke CA, Eastman A. Activation of programmed cell death (apoptosis) by cisplatin, other anticancer drugs, toxins and hyperthermia. Biochem Pharmacol 1990;40:2353–62.
36. Gunji H, Kharbanda S, Kufe D. Induction of internucleosomal DNA fragmentation in human myeloid leukemia cells by I-β-D-arabinofuranosylcytosine. Cancer Res 1991;51:741–3.
37. Griffiths GD, Leek MD, Gee DJ. The toxic plant proteins ricin and abrin induce apoptotic changes in lymphoid tissues and intestine. J Pathol 1987;151:221–9.
38. Wyllie AH. Cell death. Int Rev Cytol 1987;17(suppl):755–85.
39. Chang MP, Bramhill J, Graves S, Bonavida B, Wisnieski BJ. Internucleosomal DNA cleavage precedes diphtheria toxin-induced cytolysis. Evidence that cell lysis is not a simple consequence of translation inhibition. J Biol Chem 1989;264:15261–7.
40. Waring P. DNA fragmentation induced in macrophages by gliotoxin does not require protein synthesis and is preceded by raised inositol triphosphate levels. J Biol Chem 1990;265:14476–80.
41. McConkey DJ, Hartzell P, Duddy SK, Hakansson H, Orrenius S. 2,3,7,8-tetrachlorodibenzo-p-dioxin kills immature thymocytes by $Ca^{2+}$-mediated endonuclease activation. Science 1988a;242:256–9.
42. Umansky SR, Korol' BA, Nelipovich PA. In vivo DNA degradation in thymocytes of gamma-irradiated or hydrocortisone-treated rats. Biochim Biophys Acta 1981;656:9–17.
43. Afanas'ev VN, Korol' BA, Mantsygin YA, Nelipovich PA, Pechatnikov VA, Umansky SR. Flow cytometry and biochemical analysis of DNA degradation characteristic of two types of cell death. FEBS Lett 1986; 194:347–50.
44. Ijiri K. Apoptosis (cell death) induced in mouse bowel by 1,2-dimethylhydrazine, methylazoxymethanol acetate, and gamma-rays. Cancer Res 1989;49:6342–6.

45. Yamada T, Ohyama H. Radiation-induced interphase death of rat thymocytes is internally programmed. Int J Radiat Biol 1988;53:65–75.
46. Inouye M, Kajiwara Y, Hirayama K. Combined effects of low-level methylmercury and x-radiation on the developing mouse cerebellum. J Toxicol Environ Health 1991;33:47–56.
47. Robaye B, Mosselmans R, Fiers W, Dumont JE, Galand B. Tumor necrosis factor induces apoptosis (programmed cell death) in normal endothelial cells in vitro. Am J Pathol 1991;138:447–53.
48. Trump BF, Ginn FL. The pathogenesis of subcellular reaction to lethal injury. Methods Achiev Exp Pathol 1969;4:1–29.
49. Kerr JFR, Wyllie AH, Currie AR. Apoptosis: a basic biological phenomenon with wide-ranging implications in tissue kinetics. Br J Cancer 1972;26:239–57.
50. Wyllie AH, Kerr JFR, Currie AR. Cell death: the significance of apoptosis. Int Rev Cytol 1980;68:251–306.
51. Wyllie AH. Cell death. Int Rev Cytol 1987;17(suppl):755–85.
52. Wyllie AH, Morris RG. Hormone-induced cell death: purification of thymocytes undergoing apoptosis after glucocorticoid treatment. Am J Pathol 1982;109:78–87.
53. Walker NI, Harmon BV, Gobe GC, Kerr JFR. Patterns of cell death. Methods Achiev Exp Pathol 1988;13:18–54.
54. Morris RG, Duvall ED, Hargreaves AD, Wyllie AH. Hormone-induced cell death, II. Surface changes in thymocytes undergoing apoptosis. Am J Pathol 1984;115:426–36.
55. Stacey NH, Bishop CJ, Halliday JW, et al. Apoptosis as the mode of cell death in antibody-dependent lymphocytotoxicity. J Cell Sci 1985;74:169–79.
56. Walker NI, Gobe GC. Cell death and cell proliferation during atrophy of the rat parotid gland induced by duct obstruction. J Pathol 1987;153:333–44.
57. Wyllie AH. Cell death: a new classification separating apoptosis from necrosis. In: Bowen ID, Lockshin RA, eds. Cell death in biology and pathology. London: Chapman & Hall, 1981:9–34.
58. McConkey DJ, Hartzell P, Nicotera P, Wyllie AH, Orrenius S. Glucocorticoids activate a suicide process in thymocytes through an elevation of cytosolic $Ca^{2+}$ concentration. Arch Biochem Biophys 1989;269:365–70.
59. McConkey DJ, Hartzell P, Amador-Perez JF, Orrenius S, Jondal M. Calcium-dependent killing of immature thymocytes by stimulation via the CD3/T cell receptor complex. J Immunol 1989;143:1801–6.
60. Wyllie AH, Morris RG, Smith AL, Dunlop D. Chromatin cleavage in apoptosis: association with condensed chromatin morphology and dependence on macromolecular synthesis. J Pathol 1984;142:67–77.
61. McConkey DJ, Hartzell P, Nicotera P, Orrenius S. Calcium-activated DNA fragmentation kills immature thymocytes. FASEB J 1989;3:1843–9.
62. Kyprianou N, Isaacs JT. Activation of programmed cell death in the rat ventral prostate after castration. Endocrinology 1988;122:552–62.
63. Russell JH. Internal disintegration model of cytotoxic lymphocyte-induced target damage. Immunol Rev 1983;72:97–118.
64. Martin SJ, Mazdai G, Strain JJ, Cotter TG, Hannigan BM. Programmed cell death (apoptosis) in lymphoid and myeloid cell lines during zinc deficiency. Clin Exp Immunol 1991;83:338–43.

65. Arends MJ, Morris RG, Wyllie AH. Apoptosis. The role of the endonuclease. Am J Pathol 1990;36:593–608.
66. Gaido ML, Cidlowski JA. Identification, purification, and characterization of a calcium-dependent endonuclease (NUC18) from apoptotic rat thymocytes. NUC18 is not histone $H_2B$. J Biol Chem 1991;266:18580–5.
67. Baxter GD, Collins RJ, Harmon BV, et al. Cell death by apoptosis in acute leukemia. J Pathol 1989;158:123–9.
68. Ijiri K, Potten CS. Further studies on the response of intestinal crypt cells of different hierarchimal status to eighteen different cytotoxic drugs. Br J Cancer 1987;55:113–23.
69. Martin SJ, Bonham AM, Cotter TG. The involvement of RNA and protein synthesis in programmed cell death (apoptosis) in human leukaemia HL-60 cells. Biochem Soc Trans 1990;18:634–6.
70. Martin SJ, Lennon SV, Bonham AM, Cotter TG. Induction of apoptosis (programmed cell death) in human leukemic HL-60 cells by inhibition of RNA or protein synthesis. J Immunol 1990b;145:1859–67.
71. Cotter TG, Lennon SV, Glynn JG, Martin SJ. Cell death via apoptosis and its relationship to growth, development and differentiation of both tumour and normal cells. Anticancer Res 1990;10:1153–60.
72. Collins RJ, Harmon BV, Souvlis T, Pope JH, Kerr JFR. Effects of cycloheximide on B-chronic lymphocytic leukaemic and normal lymphocytes in vitro: induction of apoptosis. Br J Cancer 1991;64:518–22.
73. Duvall E, Wyllie AH, Morris RG. Macrophage recognition of cells undergoing programmed cell death (apoptosis). Immunology 1985;56:351–8.
74. Savill JS, Henson PM, Haslett C. Phagocytosis of aged human neutrophils by macrophages is mediated by a novel "charge-sensitive" recognition mechanism. J Clin Invest 1989;84:1518–27.
75. Savill JS, Dransfield I, Hogg N, Haslen C. Vitronectin receptor-mediated phagocytosis of cells undergoing apoptosis. Nature 1990;343:170–3.
76. Cohen JJ. Programmed cell death in the immune system. Adv Immunol 1991;50:55–85.
77. Savill J, Hogg N, Haslett C. Macrophage vitronectin receptor, CD36 and thrombospondin cooperate in recognition of neutrophils undergoing programmed cell death. Chest 1991;9(suppl 3):65.
78. Kaiser N, Edelman IS. Calcium dependence of glucocorticoid-induced lymphocytolysis. Proc Natl Acad Sci USA 1977;74:638–42.
79. Kaiser N, Edelman IS. Further studies on the role of calcium in glucocorticoid-induced lymphocytolysis. Endocrinology 1978;103:936–42.
80. McConkey DJ, Hartzell P, Orrenius S. Rapid turnover of endogenous endonuclease activity in thymocytes: effects of inhibitors of macromolecular synthesis. Arch Biochem Biophys 1990;278:284–7.
81. Smith CA, Williams GT, Kingston R, Jenkinson EJ, Owen JJT. Antibodies to CD3/T-cell receptor complex induce death by apoptosis in immature T cells in thymic cultures. Nature 1989;337:181–4.
82. Young JD, Cohn ZA, Podack ER. The ninth component of complement and the pore-forming protein (perforin 1) from cytotoxic T cells: structural, immunological and functional similarities. Science 1986;233:184–90.
83. McConkey DJ, Chow SC, Orrenius S, Jondal M. NK cell-induced cytotoxicity is dependent on a $Ca^{2+}$ increase in the target. FASEB J 1990b;4:2661–4.

84. Nicotera P, McConkey DJ, Jones DP, Orrenius S. ATP stimulates $Ca^{2+}$ uptake and increases the free $Ca^{2+}$ concentration in isolated rat liver nuclei. Proc Natl Acad Sci USA 1989;86:453–7.
85. Koike T, Martin DP, Johnson EM Jr. Role of $Ca^{2+}$ channels in the ability of membrane depolarization to prevent neuronal death induced by trophic-factor deprivation: evidence that levels of internal $Ca^{2+}$ determine nerve growth factor dependence of sympathetic ganglion cells. Proc Natl Acad Sci USA 1989;86:6421–5.
86. Fesus L, Thomaszy V, Autuori F, Ceru MP, Tarcsa E, Piacentini M. Apoptotic hepatocytes become insoluble in detergents and chaotropic agents as a result of transglutaminase action. FEBS Lett 1989;245:150–4.
87. Farber JL, Young EE. Accelerated phospholipid degradation in anoxic rat hepatocytes. Arch Biochem Biophys 1981;221:312–20.
88. Chien KR, Abrams J, Serroni A, Martin JT, Farber JL. Accelerated phospholipid degradation and associated membrane dysfunction in irreversible, ischemic liver cell injury. J Biol Chem 1978;253:4809–17.
89. Glende EA Jr, Pushpendran KC. Activation of phospholipase $A_2$ by carbon tetrachloride in isolated rat hepatocytes. Biochem Pharmacol 1986;5:3301–7.
90. Nicotera P, Hartzell P, Baldi C, Svensson S-A, Bellomo G, Orrenius S. Cystamine induces toxicity in hepatocytes through the elevation of cytosolic $Ca^{2+}$ and the stimulation of a nonlysosomal proteolytic system. J Biol Chem 1986;261:14628–35.
91. Mirabelli F, Salis A, Vairetti M, Bellomo G, Thor H, Orrenius S. Cytoskeletal alterations in human platelets exposed to oxidative stress are mediated by oxidative and $Ca^{2+}$-dependent mechanisms. Arch Biochem Biophys 1989;270:478–88.
92. Dowd DR, MacDonald PN, Komm BS, Haussler MR, Miesfeld R. Evidence for early induction of calmodulin gene expression in lymphocytes undergoing glucocorticoid-mediated apoptosis. J Biol Chem 1991;266:18423–6.
93. McConkey DJ, Hartzell P, Jondal M, Orrenius S. Inhibition of DNA fragmentation in thymocytes and isolated thymocyte nuclei by agents that stimuate protein kinase C. J Biol Chem 1989;264:13399–402.
94. McConkey DJ, Hartzell P, Chow SC, Orrenius S, Jondal M. Interleukin 1 inhibits T cell receptor-mediated apoptosis in immature thymocytes. J Biol Chem 1990a;265:3009–11.
95. Zwelling LA, Chan D, Hinds M, Mayes J, Silberman LE, Blick M. Effect of phorbol ester treatment on drug-induced topoisomerase II-mediated DNA cleavage in human leukemia cells. Cancer Res 1988;48:6625–33.
96. Kolber MA, Broschat KO, Landa-Gonzalez B. Cytochalasin B induces cellular DNA fragmentation. FASEB J 1990;4:3021–7.
97. Rao KMK. Phorbol esters and retinoids induce actin polymerization in human leukocytes. Cancer Lett 1985;28:253–62.
98. Phatak PD, Packman CH, Lichtman MA. Protein kinase C modulates actin conformation in human T lymphocytes. J Immunol 1988;141:2929–34.
99. Kizaki H, Tadakuma T, Odaka C, Muramatsu J, Ishimura Y. Activation of a suicide process of thymocytes through DNA fragmentation by calcium ionophores and phorbol esters. J Immunol 1989;143:1790–4.
100. Ojeda C, Kizaki H, Tadakuma T. T cell receptor-mediated DNA fragmentation and cell death in T cell hybridomas. J Immunol 1989;143:2120–6.

101. Pratt RM, Martin GR. Epithelial cell death and cyclic AMP increase during palatal development. Proc Natl Acad Sci USA 1975;72:874–7.
102. Cho-Chung YS. Cyclic AMP and tumor growth in vivo. In: Kellen JA, Hilf R, eds. Influences of hormones in tumour development; vol. 1. Orlando, FL: CRC Press, 1979:55–93.
103. Lanotte M, Riviere JB, Hermouet S, et al. Programmed cell death (apoptosis) is induced rapidly and with positive cooperativity by activation of cyclic adenosine monophosphate-kinase I in a myeloid leukemia cell line. J Cell Physiol 1991;146:73–80.
104. Kizaki H, Suzuki K, Tadakuma T, Ishimura Y. Adenosine receptor-mediated accumulation of cyclic AMP-induced T-lymphocyte death through internucleosomal DNA cleavage. J Biol Chem 1990;265:5280–4.
105. McConkey DJ, Orrenius S, Jondal M. Agents that elevate cAMP stimulate DNA fragmentation in thymocytes. J Immunol 1990;145:1227–30.
106. Kelley LL, Blackmore PF, Garber SE, Stewart SJ. Agents that raise cAMP in human T lymphocytes release an intracellular pool of calcium in the absence of inositol phosphate production. J Biol Chem 1990;265:17657–64.
107. Dong Y, Aronson M, Gustaffson J-A, Okret S. The mechanism of cAMP-induced glucocorticoid receptor expression: correlation to cellular glucocorticoid response. J Biol Chem 1989;264:13679–83.
108. Hege-Thorensen G, Gjone IH, Gladhaug IP, Refsnes M, Otsby E, Christoffersen T. Studies of glucocorticoid enhancement of the capacity of hepatocytes to accumulate cyclic AMP. Pharmacol Toxicol 1989;65:175–80.
109. Duke RC, Cohen JJ. IL-2 addiction: withdrawal of growth factor activates a suicide program in dependent T cells. Lymphokine Res 1986;5:289–99.
110. Sellins KS, Cohen JJ. Gene induction by gamma-irradiation leads to DNA fragmentation in lymphocytes. J Immunol 1987;139:3199–206.
111. Ucker DS, Ashwell JD, Nickas G. Activation-driven T cell death, I. Requirements for de novo transcription and translation and association with genome fragmentation. J Immunol 1989;143:3461–9.
112. Odaka C, Kizaki H, Tadakuma T. T cell receptor-mediated DNA fragmentation and cell death in T cell hybridomas. J Immunol 1990;144:2096–101.
113. Jenkinson EJ, Kingston R, Smith CA, Williams GT, Owen JJ. Antigen-induced apoptosis in developing T cells: a mechanism for negative selection of the T cell receptor repertoire. Eur J Immunol 1989;19:2175–7.
114. Lieberman MW, Verbin RS, Landay M, et al. A probable role for protein synthesis in intestinal epithelial cell damage induced in vivo by cytosine arabinoside, nitrogen mustard, or X-irradiation. Cancer Res 1970;30:942–51.
115. Cohen JJ, Smith PA. Apoptosis induced by the potassium ionophore valinomycin: potassium flux is not involved. FASEB J 1990;4:A1707.
116. Ostergaard HL, Clark WR. Evidence for multiple lytic pathways used by cytolytic T lymphocytes. J Immunol 1989;143:2120–6.
117. Sellins KS, Cohen JJ. Hyperthermia induces apoptosis in thymocytes. Radiat Res 1991;126:88–95.
118. Takano YS, Harmon BV, Kerr JFR. Apoptosis induced by mild hyperthermia in human and murine tumour cell lines: a study using electron microscopy and DNA gel electrophoresis. J Pathol 1991;163:329–36.

119. Vedeckis WV, Bradshaw HD Jr. DNA fragmentation in S49 lymphoma cells killed with glucocorticoids and other agents. Mol Cell Endocrinol 1983; 30:215–27.
120. Ijiri K. Apoptosis (cell death) induced in mouse bowel by 1,2-dimethylhydrazine, methylazoxymethanol acetate, and gamma-rays. Cancer Res 1989;49:6342–6.
121. Yuan J, Horvitz HR. The *Caenorhabditis elegans* genes ced-3 and ced-4 act cell autonomously to cause programmed cell death. Dev Biol 1990;138: 33–41.
122. Schwartz LM, Kosz L. Kay BK. Gene activation is required for developmentally programmed cell death. Proc Natl Acad Sci USA 1990;87: 6594–8.
123. Harrigan MT, Baughman G, Campbell NF, Bourgeois S. Isolation and characterization of glucocorticoid- and cyclic AMP-induced genes in T lymphocytes. Mol Cell Biol 1989;9:3438–46.
124. Piacentini M, Fesus L, Farrace MG, Ghibelli L, Piredda L, Meline G. The expression of "tissue" transglutaminase in two human cancer cell lines is related with the programmed cell death (apoptosis). Eur J Cell Biol 1991;54:2546–53.
125. Maroder M, Vacca A, Screpanti I, Petrangeli E, Frati L, Gulino A. Enhancement of c-erbA proto-oncogene expression by glucocorticoid hormones in S49.1 lymphoma cells. Biochim Biophys Acta 1989;1009:188–90.
126. Eastman-Reks SB, Vedeckis WV. Glucocorticoid inhibition of c-myc, c-myb, and c-Ki-ras expression in a mouse lymphoma cell line. Cancer Res 1986;46:2457–62.
127. Ledda-Columbano GM, Columbano A, Coni P, Faa G, Pani P. Cell deletion by apoptosis during regression of renal hyperplasia. Am J Pathol 1989; 135:657–62.
128. Buttyan R, Zakeri Z, Lockshin R, Wolgemuth D. Cascade induction of c-fos, c-myc and heat shock 70K transcripts during regression of the rat ventral prostate gland. Mol Endocrinol 1988;2:650–7.
129. Buttyan R, Olsson CA, Pintar J, et al. Induction of the TRPM-2 gene in cells undergoing programmed death. Mol Cell Biol 1989;9:3473–81.
130. Bandyke MG, Sawczuk IS, Olsson CA, Katz AE, Buttyan R. Characterization of the products of a gene expressed during androgen-programmed cell death and their potential use as a marker of urogenital injury. J Urol 1990;143:407–12.
131. Grima J, Zwain I, Lockshin RA, Bardin CW, Cheng CY. Diverse secretory patterns of clusterin by epididymis and prostate/seminal vesicles undergoing cell regression following orchiectomy. Endocrinology 1990;126:2989–97.
132. Lockshin RA, Zakeri ZF. Programmed cell death: new thoughts and relevance to aging. J Gerontol 1990;45:B135–40.
133. Vaux DL, Cory S, Adams JM. Bcl-2 gene promotes haemopoietic cell survival and cooperates with c-myc to immortalize pre-B cells. Nature 1988;335:440–2.
134. Hockenbery D, Nunez G, Milliman C, Schreiber RD, Korsmeyer SJ. Bcl-2 is an inner mitochondrial membrane protein that blocks programmed cell death. Nature 1990;348:334–6.

135. Hockenbery DM, Zutter M, Hickey W, Nahm M, Korsmeyer SJ. BCL2 protein is topographically restricted in tissues characterized by apoptotic cell death. Proc Natl Acad Sci USA 1991;88:6961–5.
136. Nunez G, London L, Hockenbery D, Alexander M, McKearn JP, Korsmeyer SJ. Deregulated Bcl-2 gene expression selectively prolongs survival of growth factor-deprived hemopoietic cell lines. J Immunol 1990;144:3602–10.
137. English HF, Kyprianou N, Isaacs JT. Relationship between DNA fragmentation and apoptosis in the programmed cell death in the rat prostate following castration. Prostate 1989;15:233–50.
138. Kyprianou N, Isaacs JT. Expression of transforming growth factor-$\beta$ in the rat ventral prostrate during castration-induced programmed cell death. Mol Endocrinol 1989;3:1515–22.
139. Kyprianou N, English HF, Davidson NE, Isaacs JT. Programmed cell death during regression of the MCF-7 human breast cancer following estrogen ablation. Cancer Res 1991;51:162–6.
140. Rotello RJ, Lieberman RC, Lepoff RB, Gerschenson LE. Characterization of uterine epithelium apoptotic cell death kinetics and regulation of progesterone and RU 486. Am J Pathol 1992;140:449–56.
141. Bardon S, Vignon F, Montcourrier P, Rochefort. Steroid receptor-mediated cytotoxicity of an antiestrogen and an antiprogestin in breast cancer cells. Cancer Res 1987;47:1441–8.
142. Rotello RJ, Lieberman RC, Purchio AF, Gerschenson LE. Coordinated regulation of apoptosis and cell proliferation by transforming growth factor $\beta 1$ in cultured uterine epithelial cells. Proc Natl Acad Sci USA 1991;88:3412–5.

# Part I

Oocyte and Cell Cycle

# 2
# Role of c-*kit* and Its Ligand in Oocyte Growth

ROSEMARY F. BACHVAROVA, KATIA MANOVA, ALAN I. PACKER, ERIC J. HUANG, AND PETER BESMER

The role of growth factors in local paracrine interactions between somatic cells within the ovary has been examined in some depth (1). However, the extent to which growth factor-based interactions between oocytes and the surrounding somatic cells of the ovary may mediate development of the follicle has only begun to be appreciated recently.

During early follicle development, growth of the oocyte proceeds in parallel with growth and proliferation of follicle cells. A priori, follicle development could be viewed as an interdependent process in which follicle cells and oocytes move through several stages, with signals exchanged sequentially to facilitate the progression of each to the next step. Alternatively, oocytes and follicle cells may be controlled independently by exogenous factors acting on each to achieve parallel development.

A third scenario is that follicle cells initiate growth by an unknown mechanism and, in turn, stimulate oocyte growth without any feedback from the oocyte to the follicle cells. However, it has recently been shown that growing oocytes release a factor that promotes proliferation of follicle cells from preantral follicles (2). In some unusual or abnormal situations, oocyte growth can proceed with incomplete development of the follicle. These include granulosa cell-deficient follicles in ovaries of LT/Sv mice (3) and follicles developing in animals treated with antigonadotropin antibodies (4). In these cases, follicle cell proliferation does not keep pace with oocyte growth during the latter half of the growth phase. Follicle cells undergo hypertrophy to become cuboidal and proliferate to maintain a single layer, but do not proceed further. Thus, although the oocyte may emit proliferative signals to the follicle cells, conditions for oocyte growth are established early in follicle development, and continued growth apparently does not require additional signals specific to this stage.

Some of the specific phenomena that could involve growth factors and growth factor receptors, or other germ cell-somatic cell interactions, are the choice between oocyte survival and atresia, the arrest of oocytes in the diplotene stage as they become surrounded by follicle cells, initiation of oocyte growth and/or release of inhibition of growth, maintenance of oocyte growth, follicle cell hypertrophy and proliferation, the retardation of oocyte growth that occurs in multilayered follicles, differentiation of follicle cells into several classes according to their position within the follicle, and acquisition of competencies to resume meiosis and undergo embryonic development that are acquired stepwise during oocyte development.

Our interest has focused on the control of oocyte growth. It has been known for some time that follicle cells have a unique relationship with oocytes in providing low molecular weight precursors and nutrients required for ongoing cell metabolism. This may be regarded as a specialization to compensate for the low surface-to-volume ratio of the large oocyte, exacerbated by the relative impermeability of the oocyte and lowered capacity to generate nucleotide triphosphates (5). When the oocyte is coupled to follicle cells via gap junctions, low molecular weight precursors are efficiently picked up by follicle cells and metabolized or passed directly to the oocyte.

Oocyte growth is, in fact, correlated with the number of follicle cells coupled to it (5). Because this close association is necessary, it has been difficult to test for additional obligatory follicle cell-oocyte interactions, such as stimulation of oocyte surface receptors by soluble or membrane-bound growth factors synthesized in follicle cells. It has been shown that coupling to other cell types, such as 3T3 cells and Sertoli cells, which should provide basic low molecular weight precursors, does not permit growth (6), suggesting that these cells are not as efficient at transferring low molecular weight molecules and/or additional specific factors (intra- or extracellular) are required.

## *W* and *Sl* Genes and Fertility

Recently it was discovered that the protooncogene c-*kit* is encoded at the *white spotting* (*W*) locus of mice. The c-*kit* encodes a tyrosine kinase receptor in the PDGF receptor family (7, 8). Mice lacking functional c-*kit* are sterile due to an almost complete absence of germ cells, in turn due to the fact that primordial germ cells generated in the embryo do not increase in number (9). These mice also lack melanocytes (they are black-eyed whites) and have a severe deficiency of red blood cells (10, 11). Mutations at a second independent locus, *steel* (*Sl*), result in a very similar phenotype, but in contrast to *W* mutations, the effects of *Sl* are not intrinsic to the affected cells; rather, they are mediated through the environment of the cells (10, 11). Complementary DNAs for the c-*kit* ligand have been cloned and shown to be encoded at the *Sl* locus (8).

A variety of alleles are available at both loci, and the phenotypes of some heterozygous mice or mice carrying mild mutations that only partially inactivate the product indicate that c-*kit* has additional functions in postnatal gonads, presumably in the germ cells. Adult mice of such genotypes may show little or no impairment of fertility in one sex, indicating that a significant number of germ cells reached the gonad in the embryo, while the other sex shows partial or complete sterility (12, 13). Most striking are $Sl/Sl^t$ mice in which ovarian follicles are arrested at the one-layered cuboidal stage in juvenile females (14).

## Expression of c-*kit* and Its Ligand in the Ovary

Initial experiments were carried out to describe the pattern of expression of c-*kit* in postnatal ovaries. Analysis of ovarian RNA or RNA from isolated oocytes and eggs on RNA blots showed high levels of expression of c-*kit* RNA (15). In situ hybridization analyses demonstrated that c-*kit* was highly expressed in all oocytes of the postnatal ovary—that is, primordial, growing, and full-grown oocytes (15) (Figs. 2.1 and 2.2).

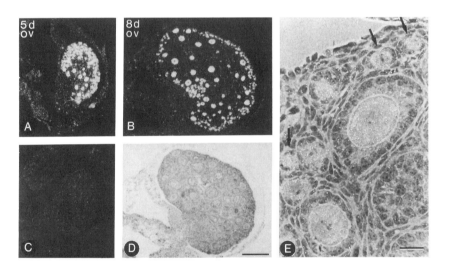

FIGURE 2.1. Expression of c-*kit* RNA in ovarian oocytes analyzed by in situ hybridization. *A and B:* Dark-field images of expression in ovary from 5-day-old and 8-day-old mice, respectively. *C:* A 5-day ovary hybridized to the sense strand probe as a control. *D:* Bright-field image of the 8-day ovary. (Scale bar = 200 μm for A–D.) *E:* High-magnification view of labeled primordial oocytes (arrows) and growing oocytes in 8-day ovary. Grains appear white. (Scale bar = 20 μm.)

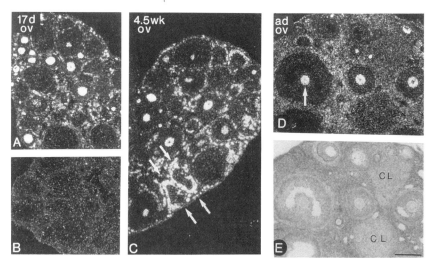

FIGURE 2.2. Expression of c-*kit* RNA in ovaries. *A:* A 17-day ovary. Oocytes and interstitial tissue are labeled. *B:* A 4.5-week ovary hybridized to the sense strand probe as a control. *C:* A 4.5-week ovary showing labeling of the oocytes and of the interstitial tissue surrounding atretic follicles (arrows). *D and E:* Dark- and bright-field image of adult ovary with a labeled oocyte (arrow) in an antral follicle. (CL = corpus luteum; scale bar = 200 μm for all panels.)

Expression of c-*kit* is initiated in the late fetus as oocytes enter the diplotene stage just before they are enclosed in primordial follicles, and c-*kit* RNA remains in ovulated eggs, but is greatly decreased in 2-cell embryos. Using an anti-c-*kit* antiserum detected by indirect immunofluorescence, the presence of c-*kit* protein was demonstrated on the surface of all oocytes; on early embryos, it declined, but was still detectable up to at least the 8-cell stage (15). Also, c-*kit* receptor has been demonstrated on the surface of ovarian oocytes by immunohistochemistry (Fig. 2.3). Thus, c-*kit* mRNA is translated in oocytes, and the mRNA may be deadenylated and move off polysomes during meiotic maturation, as do many messages (16), or translation may continue in the 1-cell embryo. After c-*kit* RNA is degraded, the protein turns over gradually and is not replaced during early development.

In light of the continuous expression of c-*kit* in oocytes, we have examined the expression pattern of the ligand in order to delineate the period of oocyte development during which kit may function (Manova et al., unpublished). RNA blots of ovarian RNA demonstrated that the ligand is expressed at all ages, but decreases between birth and 5 days of age and rises again by 12 days. Since the first cohort of developing oocytes reaches full size by about 15 days (17), this suggested a correlation between increasing expression and oocyte size. The kit-ligand is a

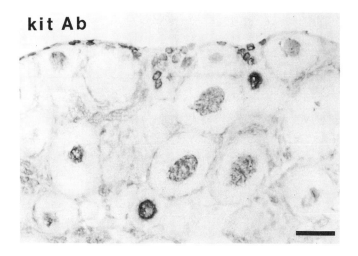

FIGURE 2.3. Immunostaining of kit in a frozen section of 19-day ovary. Anti-c-*kit* antibody was detected with a horseradish peroxidase system. Primordial and growing oocytes, some thecal cells, and interstitial tissue are stained. (Scale bar = 100 µm.)

membrane-spanning protein synthesized from two alternatively spliced forms of the message; one of these is more readily processed by proteolytic cleavage to release the soluble form (8). Both forms of the message are present in developing ovaries, with relatively more of the form that produces more resistant ligand present at birth than at later stages.

In situ hybridization and immunohistochemical analyses showed that at 0–3 days of age, expression of kit-ligand is high in medullary cords that are distinct from the rete ovarii (Figs. 2.4A, 2.4B, 2.5A, and 2.5B). Some of the expressing cells participate in formation of follicles in the central region of the ovary, and most of the follicles that have initiated growth appear to include expressing cells. By 5–8 days, significant growth of the organ has occurred, diluting the kit-ligand-expressing cells. Highly expressing medullary cords are still present, and low expression is seen in follicle cells of early-to-midgrowth-phase follicles by in situ hybridization (Figs. 2.4C and 2.4D).

Very little expression other than the medullary cords is seen by immunohistochemistry, when an antiserum specific for the membrane-bound form of the ligand is used (Fig. 2.5C). When an antiserum that can detect both membrane-bound and soluble forms of the ligand is used, considerable amounts of the kit-ligand are found within oocytes in the form of large irregular granules (shown in Figs. 2.5B for 0-day and 2.5D for 11-day ovary). These granules presumably represent uptake of the ligand by receptor-mediated endocytosis. Thus, even at the time of

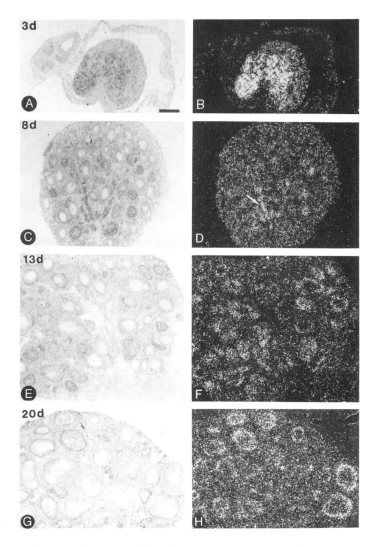

FIGURE 2.4. Expression of kit-ligand RNA in ovaries. *A and B:* A 3-day ovary. Medullary cords are labeled. *C and D:* An 8-day ovary. Medullary cords and some growing follicles are labeled. *E and F:* A 13-day ovary. Three-layered follicles are quite highly labeled. *G and H:* A 20-day ovary. Three-layered follicles and the outer layer of larger healthy follicles are labeled. (Left panels = bright field; right panels = dark field.)

minimal expression, significant amounts of ligand reach the oocyte. By 10 days (Fig. 2.5E) and increasing at 12–13 days (Figs. 2.4E and 2.4F), relatively high expression is seen in three-layered follicles accompanying the last phases of oocyte growth, when volume is increasing most dramat-

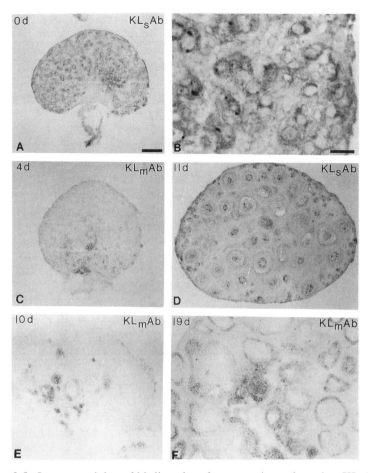

FIGURE 2.5. Immunostaining of kit-ligand on frozen sections of ovaries. $KL_sAb$ is anti-kit-ligand antiserum directed against the soluble ligand. $KL_mAb$ is anti-kit-ligand antiserum directed against a peptide in the cytoplasmic domain of the ligand and detects only the membrane-bound form. Antibodies were detected with an immunoperoxidase system. (Scale bar = 100 μm for all panels except B.) A: Stained medullary cords radiate away from the unstained rete ovarii. B: High-magnification view of A. Growing oocytes contain internal stained granules, and primordial oocytes contain small amounts. (Scale bar = 20 μm.) C: A 4-day ovary. Medullary cords are stained, and stained granules are present within growing oocytes. D: An 11-day ovary. Growing oocytes contain prominent darkly stained granules. Follicle cells of two- to three-layered follicles are lightly stained. E: A 10-day ovary. Follicle cells of two- to three-layered follicles are stained. F: A 19-day ovary. Follicle cells of two- and three-layered follicles and the outer layer of large follicles are stained.

ically. During the transition from two- or three-layered follicles with growing oocytes to multilayered and antral follicles with full-grown oocytes, expression is increasingly restricted to the outer layer of the follicle most distant from the oocyte (Figs. 2.4G, 2.4H, and 2.5F), and the stained granules within the oocyte decline. In multilayered and antral follicles, it appears that the factor does not reach the oocyte, perhaps because its diffusion is limited to the distance corresponding to about two cell layers. In adults, the same pattern of expression is observed in small growing follicles and continues in one or a few outer layers of large antral follicles.

Besides its expression in oocytes, c-*kit* is also expressed in theca cells and in interstitial tissue (15). Such expression could serve to minimize the passage of ligand between follicles or could suggest a role for the receptor in the development of these cells, mediated by ligand emanating from the outer layers of large follicles.

The pattern of expression of kit-ligand has some implications for the origin and development of somatic cells of the ovary. In perinatal ovaries, ligand expression defines a set of medullary cords distinct from the rete ovarii and also distinct from peripheral cords. It is likely that these medullary cords derive from the kit-ligand-expressing cells present in the forming gonadal ridge at embryonic day 10.5, which may be supplemented by continued invasion of cells from the mesonephric region. The non-expressing cells of the rete invade at approximately E15.5 and may also have a mesonephric origin. An outer region not expressing ligand appears by fetal day 17.5 and gradually expands, presumably due to proliferation of cells derived from the coelomic epithelium. These results support the view that follicle cells have a dual origin (18). The invasion of the rete cells appears to be correlated with increased expression of kit-ligand and, perhaps, other growth-promoting factors in medullary cords (Manova, unpublished observations). The role of the cords that express kit-ligand highly and persist up to at least 15 days of age is not known.

The pattern of expression of kit-ligand in juvenile and adult ovaries is consistent with a role in oocyte growth in several respects. First, the growth of oocytes in follicles in the medulla commences as soon as they are formed in the late fetal period, and such follicles include cells producing kit-ligand; in contrast, peripheral follicles do not grow in the perinatal period and do not express significant amounts of the ligand. The synthesis of relatively more of the membrane-bound form at this stage could help to restrict its action to the medullary region. Second, kit-ligand expression increases from low and variable in one-layered cuboidal follicles to high in three-layered follicles and, thus, is correlated with the rate of oocyte growth. Kit-ligand expression is reduced in the inner layers of follicle cells of large follicles with full-grown oocytes.

Third, the amount of kit-ligand present within the oocyte increases during oocyte growth and declines in full-grown oocytes. While we cannot rule out synthesis of the ligand within the oocyte, it is most likely that the ligand is taken up in a process mediated by the abundant kit receptor on the oocyte surface. Fourth, significant amounts of soluble kit-ligand are probably produced by follicle cells, and it is plausible that soluble ligand diffuses to the oocyte from one to three layers of follicle cells. In addition, a relatively low level of stimulation may be transmitted by the membrane-bound form on the tips of follicle cell processes that reach the oocyte through the zona pellucida.

It appears that primordial oocytes are exposed to the kit-ligand since some contain small amounts of internalized ligand, but it could not be determined whether primordial follicle cells are the source of this ligand. It is possible that a low level of the ligand promotes survival of primordial oocytes, while high levels stimulate oocyte growth. It is interesting to note that atresia of oocytes is prominent at the pachytene stage and in primordial oocytes, stages at which the receptor or ligand are reduced or absent. Follicle growth may be initiated by intrinsic or extrinsic signals to the follicle cells, which respond by hypertrophy and hyperplasia and emission of growth signals to the oocyte.

## In Vitro and Genetic Evidence for a Role of c-*kit* in the Ovary

We have initiated in vitro studies to evaluate the function of the c-*kit* receptor in oocyte development (Packer et al., unpublished). Evidence for the production of kit-ligand in follicle cells was obtained by demonstrating the survival and proliferation of c-*kit*-expressing mast cells upon coculture with follicle cells (19). In preliminary experiments we have observed significant stimulation of oocyte growth in oocyte-follicle cell cocultures after the addition of 5–100 ng/mL of kit-ligand. In addition, growth of oocytes in perinatal ovaries in organ culture or as dispersed cultures of oocytes on a monolayer of somatic cells was inhibited by the c-*kit* blocking antibody ACK2 (provided by S.-I. Nishikawa [20]).

Analysis of mice carrying the *steel panda* mutation has provided strong evidence for a role of kit-ligand in oocyte growth (Huang et al., unpublished). Homozygous $Sl^{pan}$ mice are almost completely white and slightly anemic; females are infertile, while males are fertile. Sequencing of the kit-ligand cDNA showed no change in the coding sequence, while levels of the kit-ligand RNA transcripts are decreased to about 20% of normal in several tissues. Cytological analysis showed that the level of kit-ligand is greatly decreased in perinatal gonads. Thus, $Sl^{pan}$ is a regulatory mutation that affects the level of expression of kit-ligand transcripts in some tissues and not in others.

Histological analysis of ovaries at several ages demonstrated that with a few exceptions, ovarian follicles arrest at the one-layered cuboidal

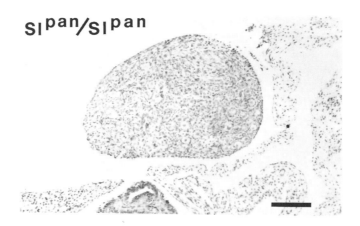

FIGURE 2.6. Section of a 4-day ovary from a $Sl^{pan}/Sl^{pan}$ mouse. In the homozygous mutant, follicles do not progress beyond the one-layered cuboidal stage shown here. (Scale bar = 100 μm.)

stage (Fig. 2.6) before significant deposition of zona pellucida. This corresponds to the stage of development reached by the most advanced oocytes at about 1 day of age in controls. These results indicate that a relatively high level of the ligand is required at this point. Whether the ligand is necessary for initiation of oocyte growth cannot be determined from these results. To assess the effect of reduced c-*kit* receptor during oocyte growth, we have examined ovaries of a female heterozygous for the $W^{42}$ mutation. In such heterozygotes c-*kit* receptor activity is predicted to be reduced to about 25% of normal, due to the formation of nonfunctional receptor heterodimers (21). The number of germ cells in the 8-day ovary was decreased, but oocyte growth and follicle development were normal (Bachvarova, unpublished). Thus, during oocyte growth the receptor is present in greater excess than is the ligand. The fact that in $Sl^{pan}/Sl^{pan}$ ovaries follicle cell growth and proliferation cease secondary to lack of oocyte development suggests that growing oocytes normally emit factors for follicle proliferation. Indeed, such an effect has been demonstrated (2).

## Conclusions

With the available evidence we can outline growth factor exchange during follicle development as follows. First, an unknown signal initiates the growth of primordial follicles and oocytes. Then, kit-ligand produced by follicle cells acts on oocytes to maintain oocyte growth accompanied by deposition of zona pellucida. While kit-ligand is necessary for oocyte growth, it may not be sufficient and may act in cooperation with other factors. The growing oocyte may, in turn, release factors promoting follicle cell proliferation and the formation of two- and three-layered follicles. Oocyte growth to full size can occur in one-layered cuboidal follicles (3, 4), suggesting that factors produced by follicle cells specifically at the two- and three-layered stages are not required. Full-grown oocytes release factors that promote follicle cell proliferation and additional factors that induce differentiation in subpopulations of antral follicles (2, 22, 23).

Kit-ligand appears to act as a growth factor for oocytes, presumably due to phosphorylation of various downstream targets (24) and activation of immediate early genes. In the testis, c-*kit* is necessary for 3–4 of the 6 programmed cell divisions of differentiating spermatogonia (20) before entry into meiosis. Kit may play a similar role during proliferation of primordial germ cells. Its action on oocytes may also be regarded as promotion of the cell cycle at a specific stage of germ cell development and differentiation. The primordial oocyte is arrested in prophase of meiosis and may require a trigger to reenter the growth phase. Kit-ligand acts to maintain the growth phase and may participate in initiation of growth as well. The program of oocyte growth presumably following from the activation of immediate early genes must include accumulation of previously unstable products (e.g., ribosomes), as well as synthesis of such new products as zona pellucida glycoproteins (25) and the transcription factor Oct-4 (26). The growing oocyte is still unable to trigger the M-phase of the cell cycle that would normally follow. The gradual acquisition of competence to resume meiosis is based on acquisition of the components necessary to produce active MPF at the appropriate time (27). There is as yet no evidence for the involvement of c-*kit* during meiotic maturation. Understanding the action of c-*kit* in promoting the important substage of the meiotic cell cycle represented by oocyte growth remains an interesting challenge.

## References

1. Carson RS, Zhang A, Hutchison LA, Herington AC, Findlay JK. Growth factors in ovarian function. J Reprod Fertil 1989;85:735–46.
2. Vanderhyden BC, Telfer EE, Eppig JJ. Mouse oocytes promote proliferation of granulosa cells from preantral and antral follicles. Biol Reprod 1992;46: 1196–204.
3. Eppig JJ. Granulosa cell deficient follicles. Differentiation 1989;12:111–20.
4. Eshkol A, Lunenfeld B, Teters H. Ovarian development in infant mice. Dependence on gonadotropic hormones. In: Butt WR, Crooke AC, Ryle M, eds. Gonadotrophins and ovarian development. Baltimore: Williams and Wilkins, 1970:249–58.
5. Schultz, R. Molecular aspects of mammalian oocyte growth and maturation. In: Rossant J, Pedersen RA, eds. Experimental approaches to mammalian

embryonic development. New York: Cambridge University Press, 1986: 195–237.
6. Buccione R, Cecconi S, Tatone C, Mangia F, Colonna R. Follicle cell regulation of mammalian oocyte growth. J Exp Zool 1987;242:351–4.
7. Qiu F, Ray P, Brown K, et al. Primary structure of c-*kit*: relationship with the CSF-1/PDGF receptor kinase family-oncogenic activation of v-*kit* involves deletion of extracellular domain and C terminus. EMBO J 1988;7:1003–11.
8. Besmer P. The *kit*-ligand encoded at the murine *steel* locus: a pleiotropic growth and differentiation factor. Curr Opin Cell Biol 1991;3:939–46.
9. Mintz B, Russell ES. Gene-induced embryological modifications of primordial germ cells in the mouse. J Exp Zool 1957;134:207–37.
10. Russell ES. Hereditary anemias of the mouse. Adv Genet 1979;20:357–459.
11. Silvers WK. The coat colors of mice. New York: Springer-Verlag, 1979.
12. Geissler EN, McFarland EC, Russell ES. Analysis of pleiotropism at the dominant white-spotting (*W*) locus of the house mouse: a description of ten new *W* alleles. Genetics 1981;97:337–61.
13. Copeland NG, Gilbert DJ, Cho BC, et al. Mast cell growth factor maps near the *steel* locus on mouse chromosome 10 and is deleted in a number of *steel* alleles. Cell 1990;63:175–83.
14. Kuroda H, Terada N, Nakayama H, Matsumoto K, Kitamura Y. Infertility due to growth arrest of ovarian follicles in $Sl/Sl^t$ mice. Dev Biol 1988;126: 71–9.
15. Manova K, Nocka K, Besmer P, Bachvarova RF. Gonadal expression of c-*kit* encoded at the *W* locus of mice. Development 1990;110:1057–69.
16. Paynton BV, Rempel R, Bachvarova R. Changes in state of adenylation and time course of degradation of maternal mRNAs during oocyte maturation and early embryonic development in the mouse. Dev Biol 1988;129:304–14.
17. Bachvarova R. Gene expression during oogenesis and oocyte development in the mammal. In: Browder LW, ed. Developmental biology, a comprehensive synthesis. New York: Plenum Press, 1985:453–523.
18. Byskov AG, Hoyer PE. Embryology of the mammalian ducts and gonads. In: Knobil E, Neill J, et al., eds. The physiology of reproduction. New York: Raven Press, 1988:265–300.
19. Fujita J, Onoue H, Ebi Y, Nakayama H, Kanakura Y, Kitamura Y. In vitro duplication and in vivo cure of mast cell-deficiency of $Sl/Sl^d$ mice by cloned 3T3 fibroblasts. Proc Nat Acad Sci USA 1988;86:2888–91.
20. Yoshinaga K, Nishikawa S, Ogawa M, et al. Role of c-*kit* in mouse spermatogenesis: identification of spermatogonia as a specific site of c-*kit* expression and function. Development 1991;113:689–99.
21. Tan JC, Nocka K, Chiu E, et al. The dominant $W^{42}$ spotting phenotype results from a missense mutation in the c-*kit* receptor kinase. Science 1990; 247:209–12.
22. Vanderhyden BC, Caron PJ, Buccione R, Eppig JJ. Developmental pattern of the secretion of cumulus expansion-enabling factor by mouse oocytes and the role of oocytes in promoting granulosa cell differentiation. Dev Biol 1990;140:307–17.
23. Salustri A, Yanagishita M, Hascall VC. Mouse oocytes regulate hyaluronic acid synthesis and mucification by FSH-stimulated cumulus cells. Dev Biol 1990;138:26–32.

24. Rottapel R, Reedijk M, Williams DE, et al. The *steel/W* transduction pathway: kit autophosphorylation and its association with a unique subset of cytoplasmic signaling proteins is induced by the *steel* factor. Mol Cell Biol 1991;11:3043–51.
25. Liang L-F, Chamow SM, Dean J. Oocyte-specific expression of mouse *Zp-2*: developmental regulation of the zona pellucida genes. Mol Cell Biol 1990;10:1507–15.
26. Scholer HR, Dressler GR, Balling R, Rohdewohld H, Gruss P. Oct-4: a germline-specific transcription factor mapping to the mouse *t*-complex. EMBO J 1990;9:2185–95.
27. Motlik J, Kubelka M. Cell-cycle aspects of growth and maturation of mammalian oocytes. Mol Reprod Dev 1990;27:366–75.

# 3

# Proteoglycan and Hyaluronic Acid Synthesis by Granulosa Cells: Regulation by an Oocyte Factor and Gonadotropins

Antonietta Salustri, Masaki Yanagishita,
Antonella Camaioni, Evelina Tirone, and
Vincent C. Hascall

*Glycosaminoglycans* are polyanionic polysaccharide chains of variable length that consist of repeating disaccharide units that contain a hexosamine and usually a negatively charged sulfate ester and/or a carboxylate group. With the exception of *hyaluronic acid* (HA), the glycosaminoglycans are covalently linked to a protein to form *proteoglycans* (PGs). These macromolecules are synthesized by a large number of different cell types and have important roles in many functional activities of cells (1).

As a consequence of antrum formation, cells in the graafian follicle separate into two primary subpopulations: cumulus and mural granulosa cells. Cumulus granulosa cells are closely associated with the oocyte to form the *cumulus cell-oocyte complex* (COC), while mural granulosa cells are organized as a pluristratified epithelium lining the antrum. The fluid that fills the antral cavity, namely, the follicular fluid, contains secretion products of the granulosa cells and components derived from the serum. Proteoglycans have been identified in the follicular fluid (2), and in vitro culture systems have established that they are synthesized by the granulosa cells and that their synthesis is regulated by gonadotropins (3–5).

Hyaluronic acid synthesis by cumulus granulosa cells dramatically increases during the preovulatory period (5, 6). We have demonstrated that the synthesis of this glycosaminoglycan is not under the exclusive control of gonadotropins. Rather, paracrine action of a soluble factor produced by the oocyte is also required (7).

In this chapter, we summarize our work to characterize the PGs and HA synthesized by granulosa cells. We focus on the most recent data concerning the role of the oocyte in regulating HA synthesis by granulosa cells.

## Chemical and Physical Properties of the PGs Synthesized by Granulosa Cells

The predominant PGs present in porcine ovarian follicular fluid are large *dermatan sulfate proteoglycans* (DS-PGs) with estimated average molecular weights in the 2–3 million range (2). A DS-PG with chemical and physical properties very similar to those described for the one isolated from porcine follicular fluid is the major PG synthesized in culture of mural granulosa cells isolated from rat graafian follicles, and it is a major secretory product that accumulates in the medium (Fig. 3.1). This indicates that these cells are the major producers of follicular fluid PGs (3). The concentration of this large DS-PG in the follicular fluid is approximately 1.5 mg/mL in small- and medium-sized follicles and 1.0 mg/mL in large follicles. Unlike the cartilage PG aggrecan, it does not interact with HA to form supramolecular aggregates. Moreover, while aggrecan is not

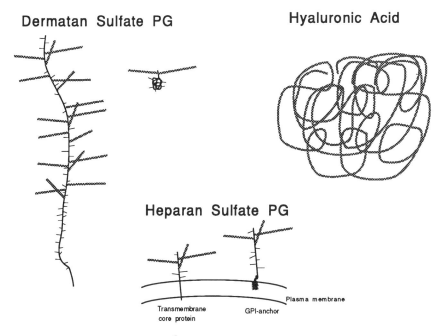

FIGURE 3.1. Schematic models of dermatan sulfate proteoglycans, hyaluronic acid, and cell-surface heparan sulfate proteoglycans synthesized by granulosa cells. Shaded lines, short thin lines, and solid lines indicate glycosaminoglycans, oligosaccharides, and core proteins, respectively. See text for detailed discussion.

significantly affected by plasmin digestion, the large follicular DS-PG is degraded by this proteolytic enzyme into dermatan sulfate-peptide fragments that contain a single glycosaminoglycan chain. Based on their molecular characteristics, it has been hypothesized that the large DS-PGs are the major determinant of the viscosity of the follicular fluid and that they contribute to antrum formation and to follicular growth and differentiation. Further, degradation of these DS-PGs by increased plasmin activity during the preovulatory period would reduce the viscosity of the fluid and facilitate the escape of the COC from the ruptured follicle.

Mural granulosa cells also produce two other distinct PG species that are primarily associated with the plasma membrane: smaller DS-PGs that have an average $M_r$ of 300,000–400,000 (8) and *heparan sulfate proteoglycans* (HS-PGs) that have an average $M_r$ of 400,000–500,000 (9) (Fig. 3.1). About 80% of the HS-PGs are intercalated in the plasma membrane (10), while about 20% are anchored to it by a glycosylphosphatidyl inositol moiety (11). The small DS-PGs are not intercalated nor anchored by glycosylphosphatidyl inositol and, hence, are associated with the cell membrane by some other mechanism, probably by interaction with other cell-surface molecules. About 70% of the cell-surface DS-PGs and HS-PGs are catabolized by endocytosis and intracellular degradation processes culminating in complete hydrolysis in lysosomes (12), while about 30% are "shed" into the culture medium, probably, in the case of the HS-PGs, after a specific proteolytic cleavage in their ectodomain (10). These processes appear to occur in vivo because follicular fluid also contains some small DS-PG and HS-PG species (3). The functions of these cell-surface-associated PGs are still unknown, but observations made with other cell types suggest possible important roles in cell adhesion, growth control and regulation of receptor functions, and cytotoxic events (1).

Mouse cumulus granulosa cells synthesize essentially the same spectrum of proteoglycans (5). The culture medium of intact COCs contains one HS-PG and two DS-PG forms with molecular properties similar to those synthesized by rat mural granulosa cells. Evidence for intracellular degradation of PGs by cumulus cells has also been reported (5).

# Gonadotropin Action on PG Synthesis by Granulosa Cells

*Follicle stimulating hormone* (FSH), *luteinizing hormone* (LH), *human chorionic gonadotropin* (hCG), and prostaglandins $E_1$ and $E_2$ stimulate PG synthesis by mural granulosa cells in vitro (4). However, while FSH elicits the same response in vivo (13), LH actually depresses PG synthesis by rat ovarian slices cultured in vitro (14). This observation suggests that direct or indirect action of LH on cell types other than granulosa cells

## 3. Proteoglycan and Hyaluronic Acid Synthesis by Granulosa Cells

present in the explants (such as surrounding thecal cells) can in turn have inhibitory effects on PG synthesis by granulosa cells. Dibutyryl cAMP and theophylline, a phosphodiesterase inhibitor, also stimulate PG synthesis (4). Since FSH, LH, hCG, and prostaglandins induce increases of cAMP levels in granulosa cells, it is likely that their action is mediated by this cyclic nucleotide. Recently, we have observed that *epidermal growth factor* (EGF) stimulates PG synthesis by mouse granulosa cells to the same level achieved by FSH and that the combination of both fails to increase it further (15). However, the stimulatory effect of FSH is increased by *insulin-like growth factor I* (IGF-I) (16). Testosterone, 17β-estradiol, and progesterone were also tested. Only testosterone consistently stimulated PG synthesis by granulosa cells (4).

FSH, dibutyryl cAMP, and EGF also increase PG synthesis by cumulus cells (5). All these substances can induce COC expansion, a phenomenon characterized by the synthesis and organization of a mucoelastic extracellular matrix (see below). However, β-xyloside treatment, which decreases the synthesis of mature PGs, does not prevent COC expansion. This suggests that PGs do not contribute significantly to this process (5). On the other hand, PGs synthesized by these cells can have a role in stabilizing the structure of the zona pellucida, the glycoprotein coat surrounding the oocyte (17).

## Effect of Gonadotropins on HA Synthesis by COCs

In most mammals, when the graafian follicle progresses to ovulation in response to a gonadotropin surge, the COC expands dramatically (18). This expansion is the result of the synthesis and organization of an extensive extracellular matrix around the cumulus cells (19). The structure of this specialized matrix is maintained during the degradation processes involved in rupture of the follicle wall at ovulation, and the expanded COCs released from the ovary are captured by the oviductal fimbria.

In all mammalian species that have been studied, the expansion of isolated cumuli can be obtained in vitro by FSH treatment. In contrast, highly purified LH and hCG fail to induce expansion of isolated mouse COCs (20). However, COC expansion in vivo is triggered by an LH surge or after hCG injection. Therefore, the LH effects on COC expansion in vivo are probably mediated by other follicular components.

The major structural macromolecule in the matrix of the expanded COC is HA that is synthesized by the cumulus cells. Net synthesis of HA during FSH-stimulated expansion of the COCs correlates directly with the accumulation of this glycosaminoglycan in the matrix and with the morphological change of the COC (Fig. 3.2). The COCs stimulated by FSH in the presence of fetal bovine serum synthesize HA at ~10 times the rate

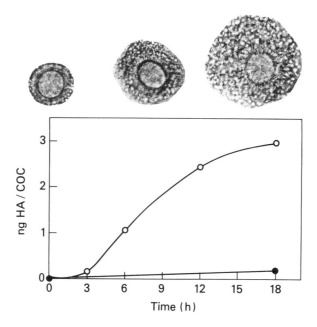

FIGURE 3.2. Time course of HA accumulation in the COC and the morphological changes during the cumulus cell expansion in vitro.

for unstimulated COCs during 18 h of treatment, the time required for full expansion in vitro, and 70%–80% of the newly synthesized HA accumulates in the extracellular matrix (5). FSH stimulation of HA synthesis is transient and is maximal between 3 and 12 h, when it increases 20–30 times the rate for unstimulated COCs. FSH appears to operate through a cAMP second-messenger system since it stimulates an increase of intracellular cAMP in the COCs (21, 22) and since cAMP derivatives, adenylate cyclase activators, and phosphodiesterase inhibitors promote HA synthesis (5, 6). EGF can also induce HA synthesis and expansion, although whether or not the effect of EGF is mediated through cAMP remains uncertain (15, 23, 24); hence, EGF exerts its effect through an intracellular pathway that differs from that for FSH.

## Effect of the Oocyte on HA Synthesis by Cumulus and Mural Granulosa Cells

It was generally thought that FSH was a sufficient stimulus to induce expansion of the COC and that the oocyte was a passive participant in this process. However, a series of experiments—in which cumulus cells and oocytes were separated by dissection and cultured either separately

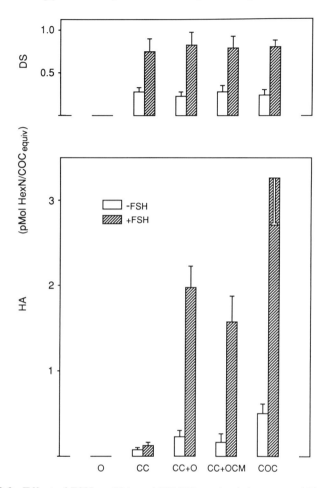

FIGURE 3.3. Effect of FSH on HA and DS-PG synthesis by oocyte (O) and cumulus cells (CC) during 18-h culture. (CC + O = coculture of cumulus cells and isolated oocytes; CC + OCM = culture of cumulus cells with oocyte-conditioned medium; COC = culture of intact cumulus cell-oocyte complexes.)

or together—demonstrated that the oocyte releases a soluble factor(s) that is necessary to induce synthesis of HA by the cumulus cells (7) (Fig. 3.3). Oocytes do not synthesize HA, and the cumulus cells synthesize only small amounts of HA when cultured in the presence of FSH and fetal bovine serum. However, when the cumulus cells are cultured in the same conditions with either denuded oocytes or with medium that was conditioned by oocytes, HA synthesis increases to levels similar to those in intact COCs, and a three-dimensional, viscoelastic matrix is formed. Growing oocytes, isolated from preantral follicles, do not support cumulus cell-mass expansion (25). Therefore, oocytes acquire the ability to synthesize and secrete the HA-synthesis stimulating factor when they are fully grown and after they become competent to resume meiosis. The oocyte factor acts either independently or downstream from the FSH-induced formation of cAMP, as indicated by the increase of cAMP level in cumulus cells cultured without oocytes (26) and by the failure of dibutyryl cAMP to increase HA synthesis in the absence of the oocyte products (7). Interestingly, in all cases, DS-PG synthesis was stimulated whenever FSH was present independent of the presence or the absence of the oocyte factor (7). Thus, HA synthesis and DS-PG synthesis are regulated independently.

Like cumulus cells, mural granulosa cells cultured with fetal bovine serum in vitro increase HA synthesis in the presence of the oocyte factor and retain most of the newly synthesized HA in the extracellular matrix (15). However, the HA synthesis response to the oocyte factor was maximal whether FSH was present or not. Most of this independence from FSH was the result of a high production of prostaglandins by these cells in culture, and prostaglandins can also induce HA synthesis by COCs (27, 28). Further, indomethacin treatment decreased the ability of mural granulosa cells to respond to the oocyte factor by more than 60% (15).

We have recently examined HA synthesis by cumulus cells and mural granulosa cells in vivo during the preovulatory period using biotinylated HA-binding region of the cartilage proteoglycan core protein as a specific histological probe (29). Immature mice were primed with pregnant mare serum gonadotropin to promote graafian follicle formation and injected 48 h later with hCG to induce progression to ovulation. At times 0, 5, and 10 h later, ovaries were isolated and sections prepared for HA staining by an avidin-peroxidase method (Fig. 3.4). At time 0 h, significant amounts of HA were not detected in either the compact COC or in the mural granulosa cell layers. By 5 h, COC expansion was apparent, and HA was abundant throughout the COC and around nearby mural granulosa cells. Staining was also apparent around antral mural granulosa cells—that is, those closest to the follicular fluid. By 10 h, just before ovulation, the COC and closely associated mural granulosa cells formed a single expanded mass that stained intensely for HA.

An ovulated mouse COC contains an average of $3070 \pm 230$ cells and $11.4 \pm 3.1$ ng of HA (29). Compact COCs isolated from graafian follicles contain an average of $940 \pm 130$ cells, and this number does not change significantly during the expansion process in vitro: $1010 \pm 120$ at full expansion. The net amount of HA synthesized in vitro per COC is $4.2 \pm 0.4$ ng. Thus, the rate of HA synthesis per cell is approximately 4 pg/cell for COCs expanded either in vivo or in vitro. The morphological and biochemical results together suggest that the larger cell number and HA content of ovulated COCs are primarily the result of inclusion of proximal mural granulosa cells that also synthesize HA in response to the oocyte factor.

3. Proteoglycan and Hyaluronic Acid Synthesis by Granulosa Cells    45

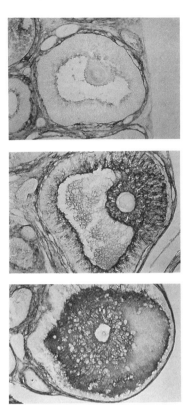

FIGURE 3.4. Localization of HA in mouse ovaries in vivo during preovulatory period. The micrographs show enlargements of individual follicles from ovaries stained with the HA-specific probe. The ovaries were isolated at times 0, 5, and 10 h (from top to bottom) after hCG injection.

The outermost layers of mural granulosa cells do not synthesize an extensive pericellular matrix during the preovulatory period and are negative for HA staining (Fig. 3.4). Differences in HA synthetic activity between mural granulosa cell subregions may reflect limited diffusion of the soluble factor released by the oocyte. This hypothesis is supported by the evidence that media conditioned by FSH-stimulated COCs, in which the oocyte is enclosed in the cumulus cell mass, have only 10%–20% of the HA stimulatory activity of media conditioned by an equal number of isolated oocytes when tested in mural granulosa cell cultures (29). In addition, medium conditioned by isolated oocytes is reduced in activity (~70%) by preincubation with isolated cumulus cells.

In an attempt to identify the oocyte factor, a number of growth factors that have been reported to affect HA synthesis in other cell systems were used to stimulate mural granulosa cell cultures (15). IGF-I, basic

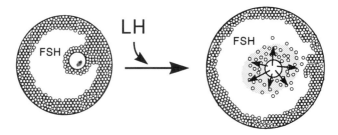

FIGURE 3.5. A model for regulation of cumulus oophorus expansion in vivo. See text for details.

fibroblast growth factor, and EGF did not induce HA synthesis. *Transforming growth factor β1* (TGFβ1), however, was effective in inducing HA synthesis to similar levels as saturating amounts of the oocyte factor. TGFβ1, like the oocyte factor, requires FSH to obtain maximal stimulation of HA synthesis by cumulus cells. However, TGFβ1 induces HA synthesis through an independent pathway since an additive effect is observed when saturating amounts of TGFβ1 and the oocyte factor(s) are used together, and an antiserum that blocked the TGFβ1 response did not inhibit the response to the oocyte factor. Therefore, the oocyte factor is not TGFβ1, and it still remains to be identified.

## Speculative Model for Regulating COC Expansion In Vivo

Paradoxically, cumulus cells do not expand in vivo until after an LH surge even though FSH is present in the follicular fluid before this surge (20). However, all the results reported in this chapter clearly demonstrate that the oocyte regulates cumulus cell response to FSH in terms of HA synthesis. Thus, we propose that cumulus expansion in vivo is positively regulated by the oocyte that synthesizes and secretes the HA stimulating factor(s) only after, and in consequence of, the LH surge (Fig. 3.5). This hypothesis is supported by the evidence that LH, acting in the follicular environment, indirectly induces functional changes in the oocyte, such as patterns of protein synthesis and meiotic resumption (see references in 30). Although morphological signs of expansion in vivo are detectable after germinal vesicle breakdown, inhibition of this process in vitro by dibutyryl cAMP does not prevent the synthesis of the oocyte factor (5–7). This indicates that these two process are independent. It follows, then, that a unique or different signal generated in the granulosa cells by LH could promote both meiotic resumption and oocyte factor production so that meiotic maturation and cumulus expansion are initiated and progress simultaneously.

*Acknowledgment.* This work was supported by CNR Grant FATMA (No. 92.00181.PF41).

# References

1. Wight TN, Heinegård DK, Hascall VC. Proteoglycans: structure and function. In: Hay E, Olsen B, eds. Cell biology of extracellular matrix. 2nd ed. New York: Plenum Press, 1991:45–78.
2. Yanagishita M, Rodbard D, Hascall VC. Isolation and characterization of proteoglycans from porcine ovarian follicular fluid. J Biol Chem 1979; 254:911–20.
3. Yanagishita M, Hascall VC. Biosynthesis of proteoglycans by rat granulosa cells cultured in vitro. J Biol Chem 1979;254:12355–64.
4. Yanagishita M, Hascall VC, Rodbard D. Biosynthesis of proteoglycans by rat granulosa cells cultured in vitro: modulation by gonadotropins, steroid hormones, prostaglandins, and cyclic nucleotide. Endocrinology 1981;109: 1641–9.
5. Salustri A, Yanagishita M, Hascall VC. Synthesis and accumulation of hyaluronic acid and proteoglycans in the mouse cumulus cell-oocyte complex during follicle-stimulating hormone-induced mucification. J Biol Chem 1989; 264:13840–7.
6. Eppig JJ. FSH stimulates hyaluronic acid synthesis by oocyte-cumulus cell complexes from mouse preovulatory follicles. Nature 1979;281:483–4.
7. Salustri A, Yanagishita M, Hascall VC. Mouse oocytes regulate hyaluronic acid synthesis and mucification by FSH-stimulated cumulus cells. Dev Biol 1990;138:26–32.
8. Yanagishita M, Hascall VC. Characterization of low buoyant density dermatan sulfate proteoglycans synthesized by rat ovarian granulosa cells in culture. J Biol Chem 1983;258:12847–56.
9. Yanagishita M, Hascall VC. Characterization of heparan sulfate proteoglycans synthesized by rat ovarian granulosa cells in culture. J Biol Chem 1983;258:12857–64.
10. Yanagishita M, Hascall VC. Proteoglycans synthesized by rat ovarian granulosa cells in culture: isolation, fractionation, and characterization of proteoglycans associated with the cell layer. J Biol Chem 1984;259:10260–9.
11. Yanagishita M, McQuillan DJ. Two forms of plasma membrane-intercalated heparan sulfate proteoglycan in rat ovarian granulosa cells. J Biol Chem 1989;264:17551–8.
12. Yanagishita M, Hascall VC. Metabolism of proteoglycans in rat ovarian granulosa cell cultures. J Biol Chem 1984;259:10270–83.
13. Mueller PL, Schreiber JR, Lucky AW, Schulman JD, Rodbard D, Ross GT. Follicle-stimulating hormone stimulates ovarian synthesis of proteoglycans in the estrogen-stimulated hypophysectomized immature female rat. Endocrinology 1978;102:824–31.
14. Gebauer H, Lindner HR, Amsterdam A. Synthesis of heparin-like glycosaminoglycans in rat ovarian slices. Biol Reprod 1978;18:35–8.
15. Salustri A, Ulisse S, Yanagishita M, Hascall VC. Hyaluronic acid synthesis by mural granulosa cells and cumulus cells in vitro is selectively stimulated by a

factor produced by oocytes and by transforming growth factor-β. J Biol Chem 1990;265:19517–23.
16. Adashi EY, Resnik CE, Svoboda ME, Van Wyk JJ, Hascall VC, Yanagishita M. Independent and synergistic actions of somatomedin-C in the stimulation of proteoglycan synthesis by cultured granulosa cells. Endocrinology 1986; 118:456–8.
17. De Felici M, Salustri A, Siracusa G. "Spontaneous" hardening of the zona pellucida of mouse oocytes during in vitro culture, 2. The effect of follicular fluid, vitamin C and glycosaminoglycans. Gamete Res 1985;12:227–35.
18. Dekel N, Hillensjo T, Kraicer PF. Maturational effects of gonadotropins on the cumulus-oocyte complex of the rat. Biol Reprod 1979;20:191–7.
19. Dekel N, Phillips DM. Maturation of the rat cumulus oophorus: a scanning electron microscopy study. Biol Reprod 1979;21:9–18.
20. Eppig JJ. Regulation of cumulus oophorus expansion by gonadotropins in vivo and in vitro. Biol Reprod 1980;23:545–52.
21. Schultz RM, Montgomery RR, Ward-Bailey PF, Eppig JJ. Regulation of oocyte maturation in the mouse: possible roles of intercellular communication, cAMP, and testosterone. Dev Biol l983;97:264–73.
22. Salustri A, Petrungaro S, De Felici M, Conti M, Siracusa G. Effect of follicle-stimulating hormone on cyclic adenosine monophosphate level and meiotic maturation in mouse cumulus cell-enclosed oocytes cultured in vitro. Biol Reprod 1985;33:797–802.
23. Downs SM, Daniel SAJ, Eppig JJ. Induction of maturation in cumulus cell-enclosed mouse oocytes by follicle-stimulating hormone and epidermal growth factor: evidence for a positive stimulus of somatic cell origin. J Exp Zool 1988;245:86–96.
24. Downs SM. Specificity of epidermal growth factor action on maturation of the murine oocyte and cumulus oophorus in vitro. Biol Reprod 1989;41:371–9.
25. Vanderhyden BC, Caron PJ, Buccione R, Eppig JJ. Developmental pattern of the secretion of cumulus expansion-enabling-factor by mouse oocytes and the role of the oocytes in promoting granulosa cell differentiation. Dev Biol 1990;14:307–17.
26. Buccione R, Vanderhyden BC, Caron PJ, Eppig JJ. FSH-induced expansion of the mouse cumulus oophorus in vitro is dependent upon a specific factor(s) secreted by the oocyte. Dev Biol 1990;138:16–25.
27. Eppig JJ. Prostaglandin $E_2$ stimulates cumulus expansion and hyaluronic acid synthesis by cumuli oophori isolated from mice. Biol Reprod 1981;25:191–5.
28. Salustri A, Petrungaro S, Siracusa G. Granulosa cells stimulate in vitro the expansion of isolated mouse cumuli oophori: involvement of prostaglandin $E_2$. Biol Reprod 1985;33:229–34.
29. Salustri A, Yanagishita M, Underhill CD, Laurent TC, Hascall VC. Localization and synthesis of hyaluronic acid in the cumulus cells and granulosa cells of the preovulatory follicle. Dev Biol 1992;151:541–51.
30. Moor RM, Crosby IM, Osborn JC. Growth and maturation of mammalian oocytes. In: In vitro fertilization and embryo transfer. London: Academic Press, 1983:39–63.

# 4

# Developmental Genetics of the Zona Pellucida

JURRIEN DEAN

The development of the mammalian oocyte and ovary serves as a focus for molecular genetic studies on cell lineage, tissue-specific gene expression, and organogenesis. The female germ cell populates the primitive gonad during the second trimester of mouse development, and their interactions with the support cells result in the formation of the ovary. After birth and during the reproductive life of the female, cohorts of oocytes grow, undergo meiotic maturation, and, following ovulation, are available for fertilization in the oviduct. The expression of the zona pellucida genes serves as a marker of germ cell growth and represents the set of oocyte-specific genes unique to mammals. These zona genes encode proteins that are secreted to form an extracellular matrix that surrounds the eggs and mediates the species-specific events of fertilization.

## Oocyte Growth and Development

Although the establishment of the germ cell lineage may occur earlier, primordial germ cells are first detected in the allantois, 7.25 *days post-coitum* (dpc) at the beginning of the second trimester of mouse gestation (1). The 15–75 germ cells present in the allantois proliferate during a remarkable migration to the gonadal ridge, and the fully colonized primitive gonad (13.5 dpc) contains 25,000 germ cells (2). By this time, in the absence of genetic material carried on the Y-chromosome, the gonad has developed morphologically into an ovary.

After entrance into the gonadal ridges, the oogonia undergo rapid and multiple rounds of mitosis that result in hundreds of thousands of cells. Over the course of several days, the majority of oogonia progress into the prophase of meiosis. Subsequent waves of apoptosis deplete the oocyte pool, and at birth (19–20 dpc), the mouse ovary contains 10,000–15,000 germ cells, almost all of which are arrested in the prophase (dictyate) of the first meiotic division (3, 4). Thereafter and throughout the reproductive life of the mouse, cohorts of oocytes enter into a 2-week growth phase, during which the surrounding granulosa cells proliferate to form secondary follicles. After the development of an antrum, the oocytes undergo meiotic maturation (5 days) and are subsequently ovulated (5, 6).

The growth phase of oogenesis is characterized by a dramatic increase in the size of oocytes (15 μm to 80 μm) as well as by the proliferation of the surrounding granulosa cells to form a mature follicle. The synthesis and secretion of the zona pellucida proteins create an extracellular matrix that serves as an interface between these two cell types and functions as a biochemical marker of oocyte growth and differentiation.

## Expression of the Zona Pellucida Genes

### Zona Gene Structure

Mouse $Zp2$ and $Zp3$ are each present in a single copy in the genome (Fig. 4.1). Mouse $Zp2$ contains 18 exons that range in size from 45 bp to 190 bp separated by 17 introns (81 to 1490 bp) and spans 12.1 kbp of DNA (7). The 8.6-kbp-long mouse $Zp3$ gene contains 8 exons ranging in size from 92 to 338 bp and has introns whose lengths are between 125 and 2320 bp (8). The genes encoding ZP2 and ZP3 are conserved among mammals. Taking cross-hybridization of nucleic acid sequences as a criteria, the degree of conservation of $Zp3$ is variable, with pig and rabbit being less related to mouse than rat, dog, cow, and human zona genes (9). The human homolog of $Zp2$ and the human and hamster homologs of $Zp3$ have been characterized. The human ZP2 gene is composed of 19 exons whose nucleic acid sequence is 70% identical to that of its mouse counterpart; it encodes a 745-amino acid protein that is 60% identical to that of its mouse counterpart (10). Each mouse, human, and hamster ZP3 gene contains 8 exons. The coding sequences of the mouse and human genes are 74% the same, and each encodes a 424-amino acid peptide that is 67% identical (11). The hamster gene encodes a 422-amino acid protein that is 81% identical to mouse ZP3 (12).

### Zona Gene Expression

The expression of the mouse zona pellucida genes is restricted to the ovary and within the ovary to oocytes (Fig. 4.2). Although ZP2 and ZP3 transcripts have not been detected in resting mouse oocytes, increasing amounts of ZP2 and ZP3 mRNAs are detected in growing oocytes. Maximum levels of the transcripts (1000 fg of ZP2 and 400 fg of ZP3) are present in oocytes that are 50 μm in diameter, representing 1% and 0.4%,

4. Developmental Genetics of the Zona Pellucida    51

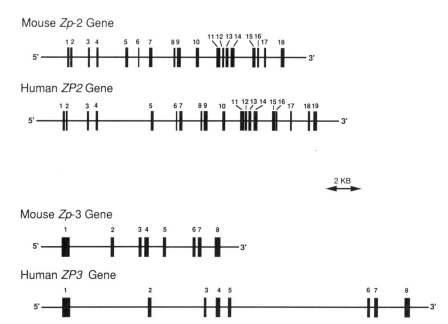

FIGURE 4.1. Exon map of mouse and human ZP2 and ZP3 genes. The top panel is a comparison of mouse *Zp2* (18 exons) and human *ZP2* (19 exons) spanning 12.1 and 13 kbp of genomic DNA, respectively, as described in references 7 and 10. The bottom panel is an alignment of mouse *Zp3* (8.6 kbp) and human *ZP3* genes (18.3 kbp), each of which contains 8 exons, but whose intron sizes vary considerably, as described in references 8 and 11.

respectively, of total poly(A)$^+$ RNA (Fig. 4.2). The molar ratio of ZP2 and ZP3 transcripts is approximately 2:1, and this ratio is maintained during the growth phase of oocyte development (7, 13). As the oocyte reaches its full size (80 μm), the amount of ZP2 and ZP3 transcripts declines, and in ovulated eggs the amount of these two transcripts is less than 5% of its peak level (7). The ZP2 and ZP3 mRNAs in ovulated eggs appear to undergo deadenylation prior to their degradation during meiotic maturation and ovulation.

If the coordinate expression of the zona genes is under the control of shared regulatory factors, the DNA binding sites of these factors may be evolutionarily conserved among mammals. A comparison of the first 300 bp upstream of the initiation site of mouse *Zp2* and human *ZP2* genes reveals that they are 70% identical. There is a TATAA box at position −31 bp and a CCAAT box at position −65 bp in the mouse gene; these elements are present at comparable positions in the human gene (7, 10). In contrast, comparison of the 5′ flanking sequences of the mouse *Zp3* and human *ZP3* genes indicates no long stretches of sequence identity.

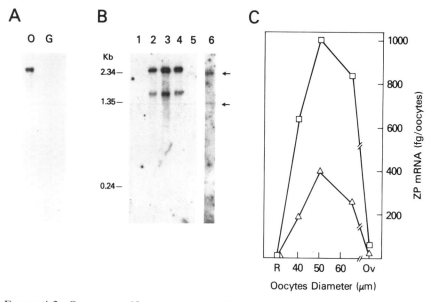

FIGURE 4.2. Oocyte-specific accumulation of mouse zona transcripts. *A:* Shown is a Northern blot of RNA from oocytes (O) and granulosa cells (G) probed with $^{32}$P-labeled *Zp2* cDNA. *B:* Shown is a Northern blot of RNA isolated from mouse oocytes or eggs probed with $^{32}$P-labeled ZP2 and ZP3 cDNAs. Lane 1: 600 resting oocytes (10–15 μm); lanes 2–4: 200 oocytes of 40-, 50-, and 65-μm diameter and ovulated eggs, respectively; lane 6: same as lane 5, but with 800 eggs exposed 2.5× longer. Arrows to the right of lane 6 indicate deadenylated ZP2 (higher) and ZP3 (lower) transcripts. *C:* Shown is accumulation of ZP2 (open square) and ZP3 (open triangle) mRNA based on a comparison of the densitometry of hybridization signals in *B* and the hybridization signal obtained using increasing amounts of synthetic ZP2 and ZP3 transcripts, as described in reference 7. (R = resting oocytes; OV = ovulated eggs.)

The TATAA box at −29 bp in the mouse *Zp3* is also present in the human homolog. Neither ZP3 gene has an identifiable CCAAT box (8, 11).

A more detailed examination of the first 300 bp upstream of four zona genes (mouse *Zp2* and *Zp3*; human ZP2 and ZP3) revealed 5 short (4–12 bp), conserved DNA sequences located at comparable distances from the transcription initiation site (14). We have demonstrated that one of these sequences, element IV (positioned approximately 200 bp upstream from the TATAA box), is necessary and sufficient for reporter gene expression driven by mouse *Zp2* and *Zp3* promoters microinjected into oocytes (Fig. 4.3). Oligonucleotides containing element IV from either *Zp2* or *Zp3* form DNA-protein complexes of identical mobility in gel retardation assays using extracts of oocytes, but not when granulosa

A. Deletion Mutations of Zp-3

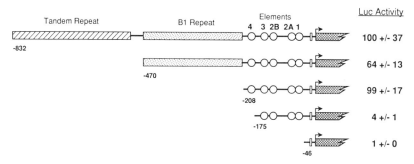

B. Mutation of Element 4 in Zp-2 and Zp-3

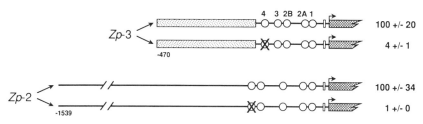

FIGURE 4.3. Mutation analysis of mouse *Zp2* and *Zp3* promoters. *A:* The top construct contains 832 bp of 5' flanking DNA sequences of *Zp3* coupled to a luciferase gene. This region contains a tandem repeat (−827 to −508 bp relative to the transcription start site); a B1 repeat (−471 to −196 bp); and 5 elements within the first 185 bp of the transcription start site (labeled 1, 2A, 2B, 3, and 4) that are conserved among human and mouse zona genes. Reporter gene activity (Luc Activity) was assayed after injection of DNA into the nuclei of growing oocytes and overnight incubation. Deletion mutants containing 470 or 208 bp indicate that no more than 208 bp of 5' flanking sequence are needed for high-level reporter gene activity. The deletion of an additional 33 bp to position 175 bp (which eliminates element IV) dramatically decreased luciferase activity. *B:* The 12 bp element IV is conserved in human and mouse *Zp2* and *Zp3* genes. A 6-bp mutation in element IV in reporter gene constructs with 470 bp of *Zp3* (top) or 1539 bp of *Zp2* (bottom) 5' flanking DNA dramatically decreased reporter gene activity, as described in reference 14.

cells, embryonic stem cells, testes, spleen, thymus, liver, kidney, or brain are used (14). The detection of the DNA-protein complex in oogenesis is coincident with the appearance of zona transcripts.

The putative transcription factor(s) identified in these experiments may contain one or more previously characterized DNA-binding proteins or may represent the first known example of an oocyte-specific transcription factor. The isolation and biochemical characterization of the zona gene activation factors will not only provide information about their structures, but will permit investigation of their functions as regulators of zona pellucida gene transcription in mouse oocytes. The concept of a common transcription factor(s) binding to element IV of the promoter region of the mouse *Zp2* and *Zp3* genes that participates in the coordinate and tissue-specific expression of the zona pellucida genes is an appealing hypothesis that can now be tested. The relatively low level of reporter gene activity in these studies (14), as well as in transgenic mice (15), suggests that additional regulatory factors are important for in vivo levels of zona gene activity.

## Biological Function of the Zona Pellucida

### Fertilization

After ejaculation into the female reproductive tract, sperm undergo a poorly understood maturation process (capacitation) before approaching the ovulated egg in the oviduct. Motile sperm pass through the enveloping cumulus oophorus, which is composed of a glycosylaminoglycan matrix and cumulus cells. They then bind to the zona pellucida that surrounds the mammalian egg (16, 17).

Solubilized zonae pellucidae from unfertilized mouse eggs (but not from 2-cell embryos) can inhibit sperm binding to ovulated eggs (18). This sperm-receptor activity of the zona has been ascribed to a class of 3.9-kd O-linked oligosaccharides on ZP3 (19). ZP2 has been implicated as a secondary sperm receptor that binds sperm only after the induction of the sperm acrosome reaction (20).

The *acrosome* is a membrane-bound organelle anteriorly located in the head of the sperm. It has been proposed that the binding of sperm to ZP3 induces a signal transduction across the sperm membrane by aggregating a sperm-specific 95-kd protein with tyrosine kinase activity (21, 22). This leads to the acrosome reaction (23) in which the sperm plasma membrane fuses with the outer acrosomal membrane, resulting in the exocytosis of the acrosomal contents. The lytic enzymes (e.g., acrosin and glycosidases) that are released, as well as some that remain associated with the inner acrosomal membrane (such as acrosin), appear to facilitate passage of the motile sperm through the zona pellucida.

Immediately after fertilization there are two major changes that prevent polyspermy: (i) a rapid electrical depolarization of the egg plasma membrane that blocks additional sperm in the perivitelline space from fusing with the egg (24), and (ii) biochemical modifications of the zona pellucida. These latter changes occur secondarily to the fusion of cytoplasmic cortical granules with the egg plasma membrane and the subsequent discharge of the granules' enzymatic contents into the perivitelline space. The release of proteinases and glycosidases modifies the zona pellucida (zona reaction), resulting in a block to additional sperm binding and inhibition of zona-bound sperm penetration (16, 24). Both ZP2 and ZP3 are modified by the zona reaction: ZP2 undergoes a proteolytic cleavage associated with the block to polyspermy (25), and ZP3 loses both its ability to induce the acrosome reaction and its sperm receptor activity (23, 26).

## Zona Proteins

The primary structure of mouse and human ZP2 and ZP3 has been deduced from full-length cDNAs representing the zona transcripts. Mouse ZP2 is composed of 713 amino acids (80,217 d), the first 34 amino acids of which are a signal peptide that directs secretion. The resultant core polypeptide (76,373 d) is incorporated into the extracellular matrix. The ZP2 amino acid sequence contains 7 possible N-linked glycosylation sites (Asn-X-Ser/Thr) and more than 100 potential O-linked glycosylation sites (7). Human ZP2 consists of a 745-amino acid protein that is 60% identical to that of its mouse counterpart (10) (Fig. 4.4).

Mouse ZP3 consists of 424 amino acids (46,307 d), including a predicted 22-amino acid signal peptide, the release of which results in the secretion of a 43,943-d protein (27). The 424-amino acid human ZP3 polypeptide is 67% identical to mouse ZP3 (11); the 422-amino acid hamster homolog is 81% identical (12). Although there is no overall similarity in the amino acid sequences of ZP2 and ZP3, they share at least one common structural motif. Each has a very hydrophobic region consisting of 23 and 26 amino acids, respectively, near the carboxyl terminus (7, 10–12, 27) (Fig. 4.4). Hydrophobic domains like these are typically present in membrane-spanning domains of proteins. The hydrophobic regions in ZP2 and ZP3 may play an important role in the intracellular trafficking of these secreted proteins or in their interactions in the extracellular matrix.

## Recombinant Zona Proteins

Given the role of the zona proteins in fertilization, there is considerable interest in defining the protein and carbohydrate domains important for specific biological functions. ZP3 serves as a particular focus because it acts as an adhesion molecule that binds sperm and then is involved in the initiation of acrosomal exocytosis. Investigations have been hindered by the difficulty in obtaining sufficient amounts of ZP3 from native sources. The cloning of cDNAs encoding mouse ZP3 (9, 27) now makes the expression of *recombinant ZP3* (rZP3) in tissue culture lines possible and represents a potential option for obtaining large amounts of ZP3. However, because glycosylation appears to be mandatory for ZP3 function, it was unclear whether recombinant ZP3 obtained from cells other

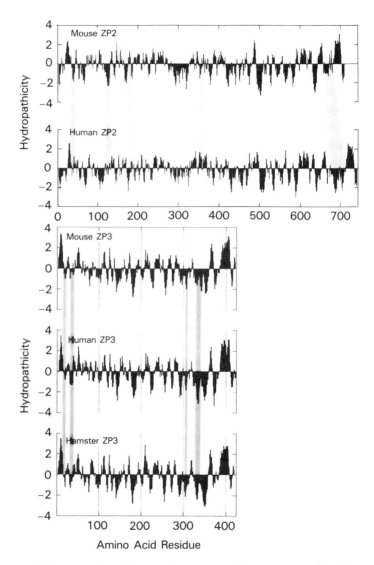

FIGURE 4.4. Conservation of mouse, hamster, and human zona pellucida proteins. Hydropathicity of polypeptide chains was determined by the Kyte and Doolittle algorithm, as described in reference 30. Shaded areas represent regions with the greatest divergence of sequence. The top panel shows the hydropathicity of ZP2 from mouse (713 amino acids) and human (745 amino acids), as described in references 7 and 10. The bottom panel shows the hydropathicity of ZP3 from mouse (424 amino acids), human (424 amino acids), and hamster (422 amino acids), as described in references 11, 12, and 27.

than oocytes would possess the necessary posttranslational modifications required for biological activity.

A full-length cDNA encoding mouse ZP3 was assembled and cloned into expression vectors that contained either a *cytomegalovirus* (CMV), or *vaccinia* (P11) promotor. Mouse L-929 cells were stably transformed with the pZP3-CMV constructs, and green monkey CV-1 cells were infected with a recombinant vaccinia virus containing ZP3. The rZP3 was affinity purified from culture media and detected on Western blots as a single 60- to 70-kd band that differed in molecular weight from native ZP3 (mean, 83 kd). Nevertheless, rZP3 is biologically active. Recombinant ZP3 decreases sperm-zona binding with a potency equivalent to that of native zona pellucida, and like native ZP3, rZP3 triggers acrosomal exocytosis in capacitated mouse sperm. Thus, rZP3 isolated from both rodent and primate cells (as well as CHO cells) appears to contain those carbohydrate and protein structures necessary for ZP3's dual role in fertilization (28). Similar results have also been obtained for F9 teratocarcinoma cells (29).

The isolation of the additional zona pellucida cDNAs in mouse (7) and human (10, 11) will permit the extension of these investigations and offers the potential of creating zona pellucida matrices in vitro. The conserved nature of the zona proteins suggests that their three-dimensional structures may be similar. Thus, more precise definition of structure-function relationships may be possible. Chimeric cDNAs that, for example, substitute the first 100 amino acids of mouse ZP3 with human sequence can be tested for their ability to induce the acrosome reaction and to inhibit sperm binding. In this manner, particular biological functions can be ascribed to different protein domains. In addition, using the cognate genes, it should be possible to create chimeric zonae in transgenic animals (e.g., mouse ZP1, mouse ZP2, and human ZP3) to further investigate the molecular definition of species-specific fertilization.

## Conclusions

The cloning of the mouse and human zona pellucida genes has provided us with biochemical markers of oocyte recruitment into the growth phase of oogenesis as well as a paradigm for investigating the mechanisms that underlie oocyte-specific gene expression. In addition, the isolation of full-length cDNAs has led to the expression of biologically active recombinant zona proteins and will facilitate the further dissection of zona protein and carbohydrate domains in fertilization and early development. The creation of chimeric (mouse-human) zonae will be useful reagents in understanding the molecular basis for species-specific fertilization.

## References

1. Ginsburg M, Snow MHL, McLaren A. Primordial germ cells in the mouse embryo during gastrulation. Development 1990;110:521-8.
2. Mintz B, Russell ES. Gene induced embryological modifications of primordial germ cells in the mouse. J Exp Zool 1957;134:207-37.
3. Jones EC, Krohn PL. The relationship between age, numbers of oocytes and fertility in virgin and multiparous mice. J Endocrinol 1961;21:469-95.
4. Baker TG. Oogenesis and ovulation. In: Austin CR, Short RV, eds. Reproduction in mammals: germ cells and fertilization. Amsterdam: Excerpta Medica, 1972:398-437.
5. Brambell FWR. The development and morphology of the gonads of the mouse, part III. Proc R Soc Lond [Biol] 1928;103:258-72.
6. Schultz RM, Wassarman PM. Biochemical studies of mammalian oogenesis: protein synthesis during oocyte growth and meiotic maturation in the mouse. J Cell Sci 1977;24:167-94.
7. Liang L-F, Chamow SM, Dean J. Oocyte-specific expression of mouse Zp-2: developmental regulation of the zona pellucida genes. Mol Cell Biol 1990;10:1507-15.
8. Chamberlin ME, Dean J. Genomic organization of a sex specific gene: the primary sperm receptor of the mouse zona pellucida. Dev Biol 1989;131:207-14.
9. Ringuette MJ, Sobieski DA, Chamow SM, Dean J. Oocyte-specific gene expression: molecular characterization of a cDNA coding for ZP-3, the sperm receptor of the mouse zona pellucida. Proc Natl Acad Sci USA 1986;83:4341-5.
10. Liang L-F, Dean J. Conservation of the mammalian secondary sperm receptor genes results in promoter function of the human homologue in heterologous mouse oocytes (submitted).
11. Chamberlin ME, Dean J. Human homolog of the mouse sperm receptor. Proc Natl Acad Sci USA 1990;87:6014-8.
12. Kinloch RA, Ruiz-Seiler B, Wassarman PM. Genomic organization and polypeptide primary structure of zona pellucida glycoprotein hZP3, the hamster sperm receptor. Dev Biol 1990;142:414-21.
13. Philpott CC, Ringuette MJ, Dean J. Oocyte-specific expression and developmental regulation of ZP3, the sperm receptor of the mouse zona pellucida. Dev Biol 1987;121:568-75.
14. Millar SE, Lader E, Liang L-F, Dean J. Oocyte-specific factors bind a conserved upstream sequence required for mouse zona pellucida promoter activity. Mol Cell Biol 1991;12:6197-204.
15. Lira SA, Kinloch RA, Mortillo S, Wassarman PM. An upstream region of the mouse ZP3 gene directs expression of firefly luciferase specifically to growing oocytes in transgenic mice. Proc Natl Acad Sci USA 1990;87:7215-9.
16. Hartmann JF, Gwatkin RB, Hutchison CF. Early contact interactions between mammalian gametes in vitro: evidence that the vitellus influences adherence between sperm and zona pellucida. Proc Natl Acad Sci USA 1972;69:2767-9.
17. Saling PM, Sowinski J, Storey BT. An ultrastructural study of epididymal mouse spermatozoa binding to zonae pellucidae in vitro: sequential relationship to the acrosome reaction. J Exp Zool 1979;209:229-38.

18. Bleil JD, Wassarman PM. Mammalian sperm-egg interaction: identification of a glycoprotein in mouse egg zonae pellucidae possessing receptor activity for sperm. Cell 1980;20:873–82.
19. Florman HM, Wassarman PM. O-linked oligosaccharides of mouse egg ZP3 account for its sperm receptor activity. Cell 1985;41:313–24.
20. Bleil JD, Greve JM, Wassarman PM. Identification of a secondary sperm receptor in the mouse egg zona pellucida: role in maintenance of binding of acrosome-reacted sperm to eggs. Dev Biol 1988;128:376–85.
21. Leyton L, Saling P. Evidence that aggregation of mouse sperm receptors by ZP3 triggers the acrosome reaction. J Cell Biol 1989;108:2163–8.
22. Leyton L, Saling P. 95 kd sperm proteins bind ZP3 and serve as tyrosine kinase substrates in response to zona binding. Cell 1989;57:1123–30.
23. Bleil JD, Wassarman PM. Sperm-egg interactions in the mouse: sequence of events and induction of the acrosome reaction by a zona pellucida glycoprotein. Dev Biol 1983;95:317–24.
24. Sato K. Polyspermy-preventing mechanisms in mouse eggs fertilized in vitro. J Exp Zool 1979;210:353–9.
25. Bleil JD, Beall CF, Wassarman PM. Mammalian sperm-egg interaction: fertilization of mouse eggs triggers modification of the major zona pellucida glycoprotein, ZP2. Dev Biol 1981;86:189–97.
26. Bleil JD, Wassarman PM. Galactose at the nonreducing terminus of O-linked oligosaccharides of mouse egg zona pellucida glycoprotein ZP3 is essential for the glycoprotein's sperm receptor activity. Proc Natl Acad Sci USA 1988;85:6778–82.
27. Ringuette MJ, Chamberlin ME, Baur AW, Sobieski DA, Dean J. Molecular analysis of cDNA coding for ZP3, a sperm binding protein of the mouse zona pellucida. Dev Biol 1988;127:287–95.
28. Beebe SJ, Leyton L, Burks D, Fuerst T, Dean J, Saling PM. Recombinant ZP3 inhibits sperm binding and induces the acrosome reaction. Dev Biol 1992;151:48–54.
29. Kinloch RA, Mortillo S, Stewart CL, Wassarman PM. Embryonal carcinoma cells transfected with ZP3 genes differentially glycosylate similar polypeptides and secrete active mouse sperm receptor. J Cell Biol 1991;115:655–64.
30. Kyte J, Doolittle RF. A simple method for displaying the hydropathic character of a protein. J Mol Biol 1982;157:105–32.

# 5
# Toward an Understanding of the Eukaryotic Cell Cycle: A Biochemical Approach

HELEN PIWNICA-WORMS, SUE ATHERTON-FESSLER,
MARGARET S. LEE, SCOTT OGG, AND LAURA L. PARKER

The eukaryotic cell cycle has emerged as an exciting field of study over the last few years due to the discovery that the mechanisms regulating it have been highly conserved throughout evolution. General principles and themes have emerged from several seemingly disparate disciplines using a variety of model systems (frogs, marine invertebrates, yeast, and mammalian tissue culture cells) and approaches (genetic, biochemical, cell biological, and physiological).

A typical somatic cell cycle consists of 5 phases: G1 (GAP period after the completion of mitosis and prior to the onset of DNA synthesis); S-phase (period of DNA synthesis); G2 (GAP period after the completion of DNA synthesis and prior to the onset of mitosis); M-phase (mitosis); and cytokinesis (reviewed in 1). The end result is the generation of two daughter cells that are equivalent both in genetic makeup and in size to the original parental cell. The cell has evolved a complex set of controls/checkpoints to ensure the accurate reproduction and dispersion of its genetic material. Failures in these control mechanisms are the basis of several human disease processes.

In yeast, a simple eukaryotic organism, there are two major control points that regulate progression through the cell cycle. There is a point in G1, denoted START, where yeast commit to enter into the cell cycle. There is also a point in late G2 prior to entry into mitosis where successful progression through the cell cycle is monitored. In contrast to yeast, somatic cells have only one point in the cell cycle (in G1) where they arrest in response to extracellular signals. This point has been denoted the *restriction* (R) point and is analogous to START in yeast (reviewed in 2). Recently, several proteins have been discovered that play key roles in regulating progression through these control points in both yeast and somatic cells. The p34$^{cdc2}$ kinase (discovered in yeast) and the mitotic cyclins (discovered in developing embryos of marine invertebrates) are two such examples.

The p34$^{cdc2}$ kinase is the human homolog of the cdc2$^+$ gene product of the fission yeast, *Schizosaccharomyces pombe*, and of the CDC28 gene product of the budding yeast, *Saccharomyces cerevisiae* (3, 4). A homologous kinase has been found in every eukaryotic species that has been investigated, including humans and plants (reviewed in 5). The p34$^{cdc2}$ kinase is a serine/threonine protein kinase whose activity is tightly regulated. While the amount of p34$^{cdc2}$ remains constant throughout the cell cycle, its activity oscillates dramatically (6–10). Kinase activity is barely detectable early in the G1 phase of the cell cycle and is maximal during mitotic metaphase. The oscillation in kinase activity involves both changes in the phosphorylation state of p34$^{cdc2}$ as well as its association with a class of proteins called the cyclins.

## Regulation of p34$^{cdc2}$ by Association with the Mitotic Cyclins

Originally identified in marine invertebrates, the mitotic cyclins are a class of proteins whose abundance oscillates as a function of the cell cycle (11). The mitotic cyclins fall into two classes, designated A and B, that can be distinguished by sequence as well as by kinetics of accumulation and degradation throughout the cell cycle (12–15). The accumulation and degradation of cyclin A precedes that of cyclin B (12–15). Association with the mitotic cyclins is a necessary step in the activation of p34$^{cdc2}$ and for entry of cells into mitosis (16, 17). Likewise, the inactivation of p34$^{cdc2}$ kinase activity and exit of cells from mitosis are dependent upon the proteolytic degradation of cyclin (18).

It is a B-type cyclin that along with p34$^{cdc2}$ comprises both *maturation promoting factor* (MPF) (19) and mammalian growth-associated histone H1 kinase (20). Cyclin A has a mitotic function and may also serve a distinct role in S-phase (21, 22). Cyclin A has the interesting property of being a part of an S-phase-specific multicomponent-protein complex that includes p107 (a protein that shares several properties with the retinoblastoma protein), E2F (a transcription factor), and p33$^{cdk2}$ (a member of the p34$^{cdc2}$ family of serine/threonine protein kinases) (23–28). In addition, cyclin A has been found twice in connection with oncogenic transformation; it associates with the adenoviral E1A oncogene (13), and it has been identified in the flanking sequences of a hepatitis B virus-integration site in a human hepatocellular carcinoma (29).

In yeast (to date) there are a single cyclin-dependent protein kinase (p34$^{cdc2}$ in fission yeast and p34$^{CDC28}$ in budding yeast) and multiple cyclins (G1 specific and mitotic specific) (30, 31). The G1 cyclins are required for passage through START, and the G2 cyclins are required for exiting out of G2 and for entry into mitosis. Thus, in yeast a single kinase (bound to different cyclins) controls both the G1/S as well as the G2/M transition.

In higher eukaryotes there are multiple cyclin-dependent protein kinases (32), as well as multiple G1 (33–36) and G2 cyclins. Cyclin A has been shown to associate with both $p34^{cdc2}$ and $p33^{cdk2}$, whereas cyclin B seems to associate uniquely with $p34^{cdc2}$ (37–39). Which G1 cyclin pairs with which kinase has not been determined. Furthermore, the intracellular targeting and substrate specificity of the various complexes are unknown at this time. Despite the complexity of higher eukaryotes, the general theme remains the same: A cyclin and a *cyclin-dependent protein kinase* (cdk) pair, the cyclin-dependent kinase is activated (sometimes after a delay due to posttranslational modifications), downstream targets are phosphorylated, and necessary signals are relayed for passage through the cell cycle.

## Regulation of $p34^{cdc2}$ by Phosphorylation

In fission yeast, $p34^{cdc2}$ is phosphorylated on tyrosine-15 and threonine-167 (40, 41). Threonine-167 phosphorylation is stimulatory, whereas phosphorylation of Tyr-15 is inhibitory to $p34^{cdc2}$ function. In higher eukaryotes, $p34^{cdc2}$ is phosphorylated on Tyr-15, Thr-161 (homologous to Thr-167 in yeast), and also on Thr-14 (42–44). In human cells the phosphorylation of $p34^{cdc2}$ fluctuates as a function of the cell cycle. $p34^{cdc2}$ is phosphorylated on threonine (Thr-14 and Thr-161) as well as tyrosine (Tyr-15) residues as cells progress from the G1 to the G2/M phases of the cell cycle and is subsequently dephosphorylated on Tyr-15 and Thr-14 prior to entry into M-phase (7, 45, 46). Dephosphorylation of $p34^{cdc2}$ at Thr-14 and Tyr-15 results in the activation of $p34^{cdc2}$ kinase activity. Threonine-14 and Tyr-15 lie within the GlyXGlyXXGly consensus sequence of the putative nucleotide binding domain of $p34^{cdc2}$. It has been proposed that phosphorylation within this motif might preclude ATP binding to $p34^{cdc2}$, thereby inhibiting the kinase activity of $p34^{cdc2}$ (40). Dephosphorylation would then restore activity to the $p34^{cdc2}$/cyclin complex by allowing the binding of ATP to the active site of the kinase.

## Regulation of $p34^{cdc2}$ at G2/M: Summary and Sequence of Events

Early in the cell cycle, $p34^{cdc2}$ exists in an underphosphorylated, monomeric form that is inactive as a histone H1 kinase (Fig. 5.1, form I). As

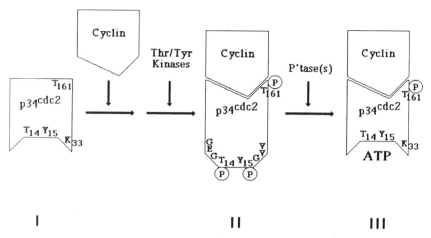

FIGURE 5.1. Regulation of human p34$^{cdc2}$ at the G2/M-phase transition. *I:* Early in the cell cycle, p34$^{cdc2}$ exists in a monomeric form that is underphosphorylated and inactive as a protein kinase. *II:* The form of p34$^{cdc2}$ that accumulates throughout G2 is bound to cyclin; is phosphorylated at Tyr-15, Thr-14, and Thr-161; and is inactive as a protein kinase. *III:* This is the mitotically active form of p34$^{cdc2}$ that lacks phosphate at Thr-14 and Tyr-15.

cells progress through the cell cycle, cyclin B accumulates and assembles with p34$^{cdc2}$ to form a complex that is enzymatically inactive but is a substrate for phosphorylation. p34$^{cdc2}$ (in complex with cyclin B) then becomes phosphorylated on both tyrosine (Tyr-15) and threonine (Thr-14 and Thr-161) residues (Fig. 5.1, form II). This is the form of the complex (denoted pre-MPF in *Xenopus* oocytes) that accumulates throughout G2. In late G2, after the completion of DNA synthesis, p34$^{cdc2}$ is dephosphorylated on both Tyr-15 and Thr-14 (Fig. 5.1, form III). Dephosphorylation results in the activation of the p34$^{cdc2}$/cyclin B complex. The activated complex phosphorylates many cellular proteins (including pp60$^{c-src}$, the lamins, c-Abl protein, and histone H1) (reviewed in 47). The end result is that cells exit out of G2 and enter into mitosis. We have determined that the wee1$^+$ kinase phosphorylates p34$^{cdc2}$ on Tyr-15, thereby inactivating the p34$^{cdc2}$/cyclin B complex, whereas the cdc25$^+$ phosphatase counteracts the effects of the wee1$^+$ kinase by dephosphorylating p34$^{cdc2}$ on Tyr-15 (see below).

## Regulation of p34$^{cdc2}$ by the wee1$^+$ and cdc25$^+$ Gene Products

Two mitotic control genes have been identified in *S. pombe* that regulate p34$^{cdc2}$ function by regulating its state of tyrosine phosphorylation (Fig.

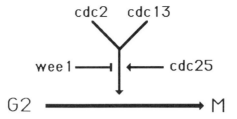

FIGURE 5.2. G2/M control in fission yeast. Several mitotic control genes have been identified through genetic screens in fission yeast. The $cdc2^+$ gene encodes the $p34^{cdc2}$ serine/threonine protein kinase; $cdc13^+$ encodes a B-type cyclin; $wee1^+$ encodes a serine/threonine and tyrosine kinase that negatively regulates the $p34^{cdc2}$/cyclin B complex; and $cdc25^+$ encodes a protein phosphatase that positively regulates the $p34^{cdc2}$/cyclin B complex.

5.2). These genes are $cdc25^+$ and $wee1^+$ (48, 49). Genetic evidence suggested that $cdc25^+$ encoded an activator of $p34^{cdc2}$, whereas $wee1^+$ encoded a negative regulator. The products of both the $wee1^+$ and the $cdc25^+$ genes act antagonistically to regulate $p34^{cdc2}$ kinase activity and thereby control the timing of entry into mitosis (49). Based on sequence comparisons with known protein kinases, $wee1^+$ was predicted to encode a serine/threonine-specific protein kinase (48–50). The cdc25 protein, on the other hand, had no obvious sequence homology to known protein kinases or phosphatases (48).

While yeast genetics is a powerful system both for identifying new genes that are involved in regulating the cell cycle and for ordering these genes in the context of existing genes in the pathway, one ultimately needs to assign functions to the proteins encoded by these new genes. Sequence analysis can provide some assistance in assigning function (i.e., similarity to transcription factors, kinases, and phosphatases). However, as will become evident below, sequence analysis cannot be used to definitively assign function. This can only be achieved by a thorough biochemical analysis of the proteins themselves.

We have taken a biochemical approach to understand how the $p34^{cdc2}$ kinase is regulated as a function of the cell cycle; in particular, we have focused our efforts on the G2/M-phase transition. Using both bacterial and baculoviral expression systems, we have overproduced several of the key cell-cycle regulatory proteins. These proteins include wild-type and mutant forms of $p34^{cdc2}$ (human), cyclins A and B (human and clam), the cdc25C gene product (human), and the $wee1^+$ gene product (fission yeast). The goal was to recreate the regulation of $p34^{cdc2}$ in vitro with purified components in order dissect the regulation of $p34^{cdc2}$ at the biochemical and molecular level (51–53). Using this approach we have made the following exciting and unexpected observations.

First, the wee1$^+$ gene product (p107$^{wee1}$ from *S. pombe*) is a tyrosine *and* a serine/threonine protein kinase (52, 53). This was a surprising finding in two regards: (i) The primary amino acid sequence of p107$^{wee1}$ predicted it to be a serine/threonine protein kinase, and (ii) at the time we obtained these results (summer of 1989), dual-specificity kinases were unprecedented. Featherstone and Russell also observed serine and tyrosine kinase activities copurifying with p107$^{wee1}$ (54). Since that time several kinases have been identified that fall within this new class of dual-specificity kinases (55).

Second, we have identified two substrates phosphorylated by p107$^{wee1}$ in vitro: p107$^{wee1}$ itself and p34$^{cdc2}$. However, p34$^{cdc2}$ must be in complex with cyclin, as monomeric p34$^{cdc2}$ is not phosphorylated by p107$^{wee1}$ in vitro. Furthermore, p107$^{wee1}$ does not detectably phosphorylate histone H1, casein, enolase, or a peptide containing Tyr-15. These results indicate that p107$^{wee1}$ has a rigid substrate specificity for the cyclin-bound form of p34$^{cdc2}$ (52, 53).

Third, the cdc25C gene product is a protein phosphatase that dephosphorylates p34$^{cdc2}$ on Tyr-15 (51). Similar conclusions were reached by several other laboratories (56–59).

Fourth, phosphorylation of p34$^{cdc2}$ on Tyr-15 in vitro by p107$^{wee1}$ ablates the kinase activity of the p34$^{cdc2}$/cyclin complex, whereas dephosphorylation of Tyr-15 by the cdc25C phosphatase activates the p34$^{cdc2}$/cyclin complex (51, 53).

## Materials and Methods

All procedures relevant to this chapter can be found in references 51–53.

## Results

### The wee1$^+$ Gene Encodes a Dual-Specificity Kinase

Based on sequence comparisons with known protein kinases, wee1$^+$ was predicted to encode a serine/threonine-specific protein kinase (49, 50). To characterize the wee1$^+$ gene product of fission yeast, we overproduced it in insect cells using a baculoviral expression system (52). The wee1$^+$ gene encodes a phosphoprotein of ~107 kd (p107$^{wee1}$) in insect cells. Both serine/threonine and tyrosine kinase activities associate with p107$^{wee1}$ in immune complex kinase assays. To determine which of these activities was intrinsic to p107$^{wee1}$, we overproduced and purified to homogeneity the kinase domain of the wee1$^+$ gene product (53). The kinase domain was produced as a 37-kd protein in insect cells, represented about 5% of total cellular protein, and was completely soluble.

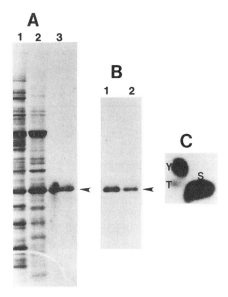

FIGURE 5.3. The wee1$^+$ gene encoding a dual-specificity kinase. A: Shown is a coomassie blue stain of p37$^{wee1}$KD at various stages of purification. Lane 1: Lysates prepared from cells overproducing p37$^{wee1}$KD were centrifuged at 100,000 × g for 45 min (20 μg); lane 2: pooled fractions from Mono Q column (10 μg); and lane 3: pooled fractions from phenyl Superose column (2 μg). B: Pooled fractions from the Mono Q column (lane 1) and the phenyl Superose column (lane 2) were immunoprecipitated with anti-p107$^{wee1}$ serum, and kinase assays were performed in vitro. Reaction products were resolved by SDS-PAGE. Arrows indicate p37$^{wee1}$KD. C: Shown is a phosphoamino acid analysis of p37$^{wee1}$KD from B, lane 2. Reprinted from Parker, Atherton-Fessler, and Piwnica-Worms (53) with permission of the National Academy of Sciences USA.

The purification scheme (Fig. 5.3A) consisted of a high-speed spin (100,000 × g, lane 1) followed by chromatography on Mono Q (lane 2) and phenyl Superose (lane 3) columns. As shown in Figure 5.3A, the 37-kd kinase domain was purified to apparent homogeneity after the phenyl Superose column (lane 3). To test for kinase activity, fractions containing p37$^{wee1}$KD were pooled after the Mono Q column (Fig. 5.3A, lane 2) or the phenyl Superose column (Fig. 5.3A, lane 3); p37$^{wee1}$KD was further purified by immunoprecipitation with anti-p107$^{wee1}$ serum, and kinase assays were performed in vitro. As shown in Figure 5.3B, a single phosphopeptide of 37 kd was detected in both cases. Phosphoamino acid analysis of p37$^{wee1}$KD from Figure 5.3B (lane 2) demonstrated that p37$^{wee1}$KD was phosphorylated primarily on serine and tyrosine residues, although low levels of phosphothreonine were also detected (Fig. 5.3C). In addition, the apparent molecular mass of p37$^{wee1}$KD by gel filtration was determined to be ~37 kd. Kinase activity cofiltered with p37$^{wee1}$KD and phosphoamino acid analysis revealed phosphotyrosine and phosphoserine (53).

These results demonstrate that p107$^{wee1}$ is a dual-specificity kinase. Recently, several kinases have been identified that fall into this category. These kinases challenge a central dogma that kinases recognize either serine/threonine residues or tyrosine residues, but not both. Two of the kinases, MCK1 (previously named YPK1) and SPK1 (60–63), were isolated from budding yeast, while three others, ERK1, ERK2 (64–66), and STY1/clk1 (67, 68), were isolated from mammalian systems. Thus, dual-specificity kinases appear to be ubiquitous in eukaryotes. To date, no tyrosine-specific protein kinase has been isolated from yeast.

## Cdc25$^+$ Encodes a Protein Phosphatase

Whereas wee1$^+$ encodes a negative regulator of the cell cycle, genetic evidence suggested that cdc25$^+$ encodes a positive regulator of the cell cycle. In order to characterize the biochemical activity associated with the cdc25 protein and to elucidate the contribution made by cdc25$^+$ to the regulation of p34$^{cdc2}$, we have overproduced full-length as well as deletion mutants of the cdc25C protein (human homolog) in bacteria (51).

To facilitate the purification of the human cdc25C gene product, a bacterial expression vector was constructed that expressed the full-length cdc25C gene product (as well as deletion mutants) as a fusion protein with the *S. japonicus* glutathione S-transferase gene. As seen in Figure 5.4A (lane 2), the majority of the 80-kd cdc25C fusion protein (p80GST-cdc25C) was present in the insoluble fraction of the bacterial lysate; however, the soluble fraction (~1%) was easily purified by affinity chromatography on glutathione coupled to agarose. As seen in Figure 5.4A (lane 1), *glutathione S-transferase* (GST) migrated with a molecular weight of approximately 26 kd. Also evident in lanes 1 and 2 is an endogenous bacterial protein of approximately 70 kd (species 1) that copurified with GST and p80GST-cdc25C. Another bacterial protein of approximately 60 kd (species 2, lane 2) copurified with p80GST-cdc25C. Species 3 was generated during the purification of p80GST-cdc25C, was recognized by an antibody specific for the cdc25C protein, and thus is likely to be a degradation product of p80GST-cdc25C (data not shown). Smaller species of 27–30 kd were also detected and may represent readthrough products of GST. Copurifying bacterial proteins with similar molecular weights to those seen in Figure 5.4A have been reported by others using this system (69).

Genetics indicated that cdc25$^+$ was a positive regulator of the cell cycle that acted in opposition to wee1$^+$. Since wee1$^+$ encoded a protein kinase, one model that could be put forth is that cdc25$^+$ encodes a protein phosphatase that reverses the effects of the wee1$^+$ gene product. In an attempt to establish a biochemically pure assay system for determining

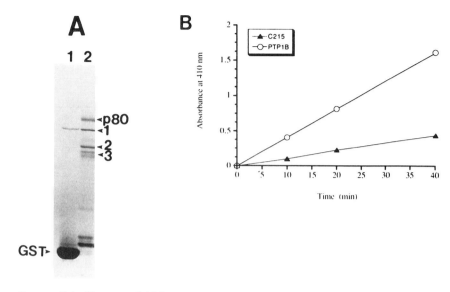

FIGURE 5.4. Human cdc25C gene encoding a protein phosphatase. *A:* Lysates prepared from bacteria expressing either the glutathione S-transferase leader sequence from pGEX-2T (lane 1) or the cdc25C-fusion protein from pML25 (lane 2) were prepared and incubated with glutathione-agarose beads. The beads were washed, and the bound proteins were eluted by boiling in SDS-sample buffer. Proteins were resolved by SDS-PAGE on a 12% gel and visualized by Coomassie blue staining. Species 1 and 2 are copurifying bacterial proteins, and species 3 is a breakdown product of the cdc25C-fusion protein. *B:* The C-terminal domain (C215) of the cdc25C protein (2 µg) and placental phosphatase 1B (PTP1B) (0.63 µg) were incubated with PNPP. At the times indicated the reactions were terminated, and absorbance at 410 mm was measured. Reprinted from Lee, Ogg, Xu, et al. (51) with permission of the American Society of Cell Biology.

whether cdc25C protein was indeed a phosphatase, we tested the ability of *p-nitrophenyl phosphate* (PNPP, a commonly used artificial substrate for monitoring tyrosine-specific protein phosphatase activity) to be hydrolyzed by recombinant cdc25C protein. In this experiment, the C-terminal domain of the cdc25C protein (denoted C215), rather than full-length cdc25 protein, was used. As shown in Figure 5.4B, PNPP was hydrolyzed at a rate of nearly 10% that of PTP1B, indicating that the activity associated with the cdc25C protein was a biochemically significant activity. In addition, we utilized affinity-purifed bacterially derived cdc25C protein and an artificial substrate (PNPP), thus ruling out the possibility that a tyrosine phosphatase other than cdc25C itself was responsible for the activity. The specific activity of C215C was calculated to be about 300 units/mg of recombinant protein compared with 3600 units/mg for bacterially produced PTP1B. (Specific activity is defined as pmole of PNPP hydrolyzed per min per mg of recombinant protein.) (51). These results indicate that the phosphatase activity is intrinsic to the cdc25C protein.

The cdc25C protein lacks obvious homology to known protein phosphatases, although Moreno and Nurse (70) recently noted homology between the *S. pombe* cdc25 protein and VH1, a phosphatase encoded by vaccinia virus that is capable of hydrolyzing phosphoserine and phosphotyrosine (71). The cdc25C protein contains a motif (HCXAGXXR) within its C-terminus that is conserved in the active site of all known tyrosine-specific protein phosphatases. Mutation of the cysteine residue within this motif ablates the phosphatase activity of VH1 (71). Mutation of this cysteine residue in homologs of $cdc25^+$ also ablates phosphatase activity (56–58).

## *Regulation of the $p34^{cdc2}$/Cyclin B Complex by the $wee1^+$ and $cdc25^+$ Gene Products*

In both fission yeast and higher eukaryotes, tyrosine phosphorylation inhibits the biochemical and biological properties of the $p34^{cdc2}$/cyclin B complex. The $wee1^+$ and $cdc25^+$ gene products have been implicated in regulating $p34^{cdc2}$ via tyrosine phosphorylation and dephosphorylation, respectively. However, a direct biochemical confirmation of this model has been lacking. We have developed a system to study the interactions between the $p34^{cdc2}$/cyclin B complex and the $wee1^+$ and $cdc25^+$ proteins in vitro. We have overproduced the $wee1^+$ and human cyclin B proteins in insect cells as fusions with GST (53). Both proteins are easily purified using glutathione agarose beads as an affinity reagent. In addition, large quantities of $p34^{cdc2}$/cyclin B complex can be isolated by coproducing $p34^{cdc2}$ with GST-cyclin B in insect cells. Using this system, we recently demonstrated that $p34^{cdc2}$ is phosphorylated by $p107^{wee1}$ in vitro only when it is bound to cyclin (53). The phosphorylation occurs on Tyr-15 and inhibits the kinase activity of the complex. To examine the effects of the cdc25C phosphatase in this system, we overproduced the catalytic domain of the cdc25C phosphatase in bacteria as a fusion with GST (GST-C215C) and tested for its ability to dephosphorylate and activate $p34^{cdc2}$ (51).

As shown in Figure 5.5A (lane 5), $p34^{cdc2}$ was phosphorylated upon incubation with GST-$p107^{wee1}$ in vitro. $p34^{cdc2}$ was not detectably phosphorylated in the absence of GST-$p107^{wee1}$ (lane 3) nor in the presence of GST (lane 4). The addition of bacterially derived cdc25C protein resulted in the dephosphorylation of $p34^{cdc2}$ (lane 6), and this cdc25C-dependent dephosphorylation was blocked by sodium orthovanadate (lane 7). The cdc25C phosphatase appeared specific for $p34^{cdc2}$, as neither cyclin B nor GST-$p107^{wee1}$ were detectably dephosphorylated under these conditions. Phosphoamino acid analysis of $p34^{cdc2}$ phosphorylated by GST-$p107^{wee1}$

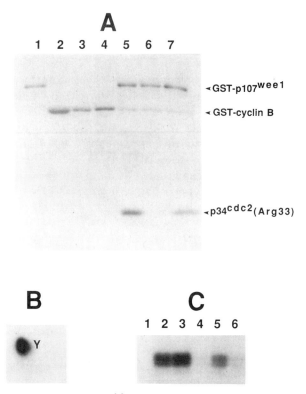

FIGURE 5.5. Regulation of p34$^{cdc2}$/cyclin B by wee1$^+$ and cdc25C$^+$ proteins in vitro. *A:* Insect cells were infected with viruses encoding GST, GST-cyclin B, or GST-p107$^{wee1}$ or were coinfected with viruses encoding GST-cyclin B and p34$^{cdc2}$(Arg 33). Lysates were prepared, proteins were precipitated with glutathione agarose beads, and kinase reactions were performed in the presence of gamma $^{32}$P-labeled ATP. Kinase reactions were washed; then phosphatase assays were performed in the presence of either phosphatase buffer alone (lanes 1–5) or with phosphatase buffer containing the catalytic domain of the cdc25C protein in the absence (lane 6) or in the presence of 2 mM sodium orthovanadate (lane 7). Reactions were stopped by boiling in SDS-sample buffer, and proteins were resolved by SDS-PAGE. Precipitated lysates were as follows: GST-p107$^{wee1}$ (lane 1); GST-cyclin B (lane 2); p34$^{cdc2}$(Arg 33)/GST-cyclin B (lane 3); p34$^{cdc2}$(Arg 33)/GST-cyclin B mixed with GST (lane 4); and p34$^{cdc2}$(Arg 33)/GST-cyclin B mixed with GST-p107$^{wee1}$ (lanes 5–7). *B:* Two-dimensional phosphoamino acid analysis of p34$^{cdc2}$(Arg 33) from *A* (lane 5). (Y = phosphotyrosine.) *C:* Insect cells were infected with viruses encoding either GST or GST-p107$^{wee1}$ or were coinfected with viruses encoding GST-cyclin B and wild-type p34$^{cdc2}$. Lysates were prepared, proteins were precipitated with glutathione agarose beads, and phosphorylation reactions were performed in the presence of 1 mM unlabeled ATP. Samples were washed, and phosphatase assays were performed in the presence of phosphatase buffer (lanes 1–4) or phosphatase buffer containing the catalytic domain of the cdc25C phosphatase in the absence (lane 5) or in the presence of 2 mM sodium orthovanadate (lane 6). Reactions were washed, and histone H1 kinase assays were performed. Recombinant cdc25C protein was assayed for histone H1 kinase activity (lane 1). Precipitated insect cell lysates were as follows: p34$^{cdc2}$/GST-cyclin B (lane 2); p34$^{cdc2}$/GST-cyclin B mixed with GST (lane 3); and p34$^{cdc2}$/GST-cyclin B mixed with GST-p107$^{wee1}$ (lanes 4–6).

in vitro revealed only phosphotyrosine (Fig. 5.5B), and phosphotryptic maps identified a single phosphopeptide that was identical to the Tyr-15 containing phosphotryptic peptide of p34$^{cdc2}$ (data not shown). A kinase-deficient mutant of p34$^{cdc2}$ (p34$^{cdc2}$ [Arg 33], where Lys 33 was replaced with Arg) was assayed in this experiment to reduce background phosphorylation due to the activity of the p34$^{cdc2}$/cyclin complex itself. Thus, the low level of GST-cyclin B phosphorylation evident in lanes 2–7 is due to the coprecipitation of a host kinase with GST-cyclin B.

To examine the functional consequences of tyrosine phosphorylation, histone H1 kinase assays were performed (Fig. 5.5C). In this case, wild-type p34$^{cdc2}$/GST-cyclin B complexes were used. As seen in lane 4, phosphorylation of the p34$^{cdc2}$/GST-cyclin B complex by GST-p107$^{wee1}$ in vitro ablated the kinase activity of the complex. Addition of the catalytic domain of the cdc25C phosphatase reactivated the histone H1 kinase activity to 52% of the original level (lane 5), and sodium orthovanadate inhibited the cdc25C-dependent activation (lane 6). Preparations of the cdc25C protein lacked detectable histone H1 kinase activity (lane 1).

## Discussion

The biochemical studies summarized above demonstrate that wee1$^+$ and cdc25$^+$ function as mitotic control genes by directly regulating p34$^{cdc2}$ kinase activity. These studies confirm certain predictions made from genetic studies conducted in fission yeast. Genetics indicated that wee1$^+$ was a negative regulator of mitosis and that cdc25$^+$ functioned antagonistically with wee1$^+$ as a positive regulator of mitosis. The biochemistry reported here demonstrates that the wee1$^+$ kinase negatively regulates the entry of cells into mitosis by phosphorylating p34$^{cdc2}$ on Tyr-15, an inhibitory modification. The cdc25$^+$ phosphatase acts in opposition to the wee1$^+$ kinase by dephosphorylating p34$^{cdc2}$ on Tyr-15, thereby activating it.

Although these studies have provided a more comprehensive view of how the eukaryotic cell cycle is regulated, several important questions remain to be addressed. For example, how does the addition of growth factors to the plasma membrane of a cell become translated as a signal for that cell to commence cell division? The ultimate goal of this question is to delineate the sequence of events set in motion from the time a cell receives a growth stimulatory signal to the time when that cell has duplicated and distributed its genetic material equally to two daughter cells. By working in the forward direction (from growth factor to growth factor receptor to primary substrates/targets of phosphorylation) as well as backwards (from p34$^{cdc2}$), one hopes eventually to see a meeting somewhere in the middle. One can work backwards by asking the following questions (Fig. 5.6).

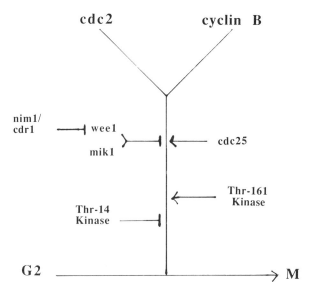

FIGURE 5.6. Summary of the regulation of the p34$^{cdc2}$/cyclin B complex at the G2/M-phase transition. See text for an explanation of the regulators.

How is the wee1$^+$ kinase regulated as a function of the cell cycle? The p107$^{wee1}$ is a phosphoprotein and thus may itself be regulated by phosphorylation. In fact, genetics has identified another gene, cdr1$^+$/nim1$^+$, that is placed upstream of wee1$^+$ and is a positive regulator of mitosis (72, 73). By sequence cdr1$^+$/nim1$^+$ is predicted to encode a protein kinase. One model currently being tested is that cdr1$^+$/nim1$^+$ directly phosphorylates p107$^{wee1}$, thereby inhibiting it. If this model proves correct, one can then ask what regulates cdr1$^+$/nim1$^+$ and continue to work through the pathway this way.

How do kinases other than that encoded by wee1$^+$ contribute to the regulation of Tyr-15 phosphorylation? We have identified p107$^{wee1}$ as one tyrosine kinase that regulates p34$^{cdc2}$, yet others have shown that deletion of the wee1$^+$ gene from fission yeast does not detectably alter the levels of p34$^{cdc2}$ tyrosine phosphorylation (74). These conflicting results can be resolved if one proposes redundancy and argues for the presence of one or more tyrosine kinases in fission yeast that regulate p34$^{cdc2}$. Indeed, genetic screens in S. pombe have identified a homolog of wee1$^+$, the mik1$^+$ gene (75). A double deletion of both wee1$^+$ and mik1$^+$ results in a loss in p34$^{cdc2}$ tyrosine phosphorylation and is lethal. The mik1$^+$ gene encodes a putative protein kinase with 48% amino acid identity to the wee1$^+$ gene product over the catalytic domain. Based on results obtained for p107$^{wee1}$, it has been assumed that mik1$^+$ encodes a tyrosine kinase (or dual-function kinase) that directly regulates the p34$^{cdc2}$ kinase by tyrosine phosphorylation (76). However, there are no biochemical data to support this model.

How is the cdc25$^+$ phosphatase—there are 3 human genes identified to date (76)—regulated as a function of the cell cycle? An inactive form of the p34$^{cdc2}$/cyclin B complex accumulates throughout G2. Once the cell is prepared to enter into mitosis (i.e., the DNA is intact and fully replicated), the cdc25 phosphatase dephosphorylates the complex and activates it. Thus, it is critical that the cdc25 phosphatase not gain access to the complex prior to the appropriate time in the cell cycle. Levels of the cdc25C phosphatase have been shown to be constant throughout the cell cycle (in higher eukaryotes [77]); thus, either the cdc25 phosphatase is held in an inactive state or the phosphatase is sequestered from the complex until the appropriate time. The cdc25 phosphatase is a phosphoprotein, and its state of phosphorylation varies as a function of the cell cycle. Thus, the activity of the cdc25 phosphatase may be directly regulated by its state of phosphorylation. Experiments designed to identify the kinases and phosphatases that utilize the cdc25C phosphatase as a substrate are currently under way. Once these kinases and phosphatases are identified, one can ask how they are regulated and thus continue up the pathway.

What are the threonine kinases that phosphorylate p34$^{cdc2}$ as a function of the cell cycle? In higher eukaryotes, p34$^{cdc2}$ is phosphorylated on Thr-14 as well as on Tyr-15 (in fission yeast Thr-14 phosphorylation has not been detected) (42). Both residues are located within the putative ATP binding site of p34$^{cdc2}$, and phosphorylation within this domain is inhibitory to p34$^{cdc2}$ kinase activity (40). Because p107$^{wee1}$ is a serine/threonine and tyrosine kinase, it is reasonable to predict that p107$^{wee1}$ would phosphorylate p34$^{cdc2}$ on Thr-14 as well as on Tyr-15, yet we have not observed any threonine phosphorylation of p34$^{cdc2}$ by p107$^{wee1}$. However, our studies have been carried out with human p34$^{cdc2}$ and S. pombe p107$^{wee1}$. It is possible that the human homolog of p107$^{wee1}$ in similar assays would catalyze the phosphorylation of human p34$^{cdc2}$ on both Thr-14 and Tyr-15. It is also possible that the phosphorylation of p34$^{cdc2}$ on Thr-14 is catalyzed by a kinase that has yet to be identified.

In higher eukaryotes, Thr-161 is also a site of regulatory phosphorylation. Although Thr-161 of p34$^{cdc2}$ aligns with the autophosphorylation site of cAMP-dependent protein kinase, the phosphorylation of Thr-161 does not appear to occur by an intramolecular route in the case of p34$^{cdc2}$. The identity of the Thr-161 kinase and the elucidation of its regulation are expected to contribute greatly to our understanding of cell-cycle control.

What are the critical substrates of the activated cyclin/cdk complexes, and how is the activated kinase specifically targeted to these substrates? The cyclin A/p33$^{cdk2}$ complex has been found in an S-phase-specific ternary complex with the RB-like protein p107 and the transcription factor E2F (23–28). Thus, both p107 and E2F are potential substrates of the activated $p33^{cdk2}$, and their activity, in turn, may be regulated by phosphorylation. Whether p107 and E2F are indeed substrates of the cyclin A/$p33^{cdck2}$ complex and how their phosphorylation regulates S-phase-specific functions remain to be elucidated.

The cyclin B/$p34^{cdc2}$ kinase appears to be a fairly promiscuous kinase and phosphorylates many cellular substrates, some that are structural (histone H1, the lamins, and HMG I) and others that are regulatory ($pp60^{c-src}$, c-Abl protein, and SWI5) (reviewed in 47). It is still unclear at this time how the phosphorylation of these downstream targets is eventually translated into a signal for cells to exit out of G2 and enter into mitosis.

*Acknowledgments.* This work was supported by NIH Grant GM-47017 to H.P-W and NIH Public Health Service Award CA-08894-01A1 to L.L.P. H.P-W is a Pew Scholar in the Biomedical Sciences.

## *References*

1. Pardee AB. G1 events and regulation of cell proliferation. Science 1989; 246:603–8.
2. Murray AW, Kirschner MW. Dominoes and clocks: the union of two views of the cell cycle. Science 1989;246:614–21.
3. Beach D, Durkacz B, Nurse P. Functional homologous cell cycle control genes in budding and fission yeast. Nature 1982;300:706–9.
4. Lee M, Nurse P. Complementation used to clone a human homolog of the fission yeast cell cycle control gene cdc2. Nature 1987;327:31–5.
5. Nurse P. Universal control mechanism regulating onset of M-phase. Nature 1990;344:503–7.
6. Booher R, Alfa E, Hyams J, Beach D. The fission yeast cdc2/cdc13/suc1 protein kinase: regulation of catalytic activity and nuclear localization. Cell 1989;58:485–97.
7. Gautier J, Matsukawa T, Nurse P, Maller J. Dephosphorylation and activation of *Xenopus* p34cdc2 protein kinase during the cell cycle. Nature 1989;339:626–9.
8. Labbe JC, Lee MG, Nurse P, Picard A, Doree M. Activation at M-phase of a protein kinase encoded by a starfish homologue of the cell cycle control gene cdc2. Nature 1988;335:251–4.
9. Draetta G, Beach D. Activation of cdc2 protein kinase during mitosis in human cells: cell cycle-dependent phosphorylation and subunit rearrangement. Cell 1988;54:17–26.
10. Moreno S, Hayles J, PN. Regulation of p34cdc2 protein kinase during mitosis. Cell 1989;58:361–72.
11. Evans T, Rosenthal ET, Youngblom J, Distel D, Hunt T. Cyclin A protein specified by maternal mRNA in sea urchin eggs that is destroyed at each cleavage division. Cell 1983;33:389–96.

12. Pines J, Hunter T. Isolation of a human cyclin cDNA: evidence for cyclin mRNA and protein regulation in the cell cycle and for interaction with p34cdc2. Cell 1989;58:833–46.
13. Pines J, Hunter T. Human cyclin A is adenovirus E1A-associated protein p60 and behaves differently from cyclin B. Nature 1990;346:760–3.
14. Swenson K, Farrell K, Ruderman J. The clam embryo protein cyclin A induces entry into M phase and the resumption of meiosis in *Xenopus* oocytes. Cell 1986;47:861–70.
15. Westendorf J, Swenson K, Ruderman J. The role of cyclin B in meiosis 1. J Cell Biol 1989;108:1431–43.
16. Minshull J, Golsteyn R, Hill CS, Hunt T. The A- and B-type cyclin associated cdc2 kinases in *Xenopus* turn on and off at different times in the cell cycle. EMBO J 1990;9:2865–75.
17. Murray AW, Kirschner MW. Cyclin synthesis drives the early embryonic cell cycle. Nature 1989;339:275–80.
18. Murray AW, Solomon MJ, Kirschner MW. The role of cyclin synthesis and degradation in the control of maturation promoting factor activity. Nature 1989;339:280–6.
19. Gautier J, Minshull J, Lohka M, Glotzer M, Hunt T, Maller JL. Cyclin is a component of maturation-promoting factor from *Xenopus*. Cell 1990;60:487–94.
20. Langan TA, Gautier J, Lohka M, et al. Mammalian growth-associated H1 histone kinase: a homolog of cdc2+/CDC28 protein kinases controlling mitotic entry into yeast and frog cells. Mol Cell Biol 1989;9:3860–8.
21. Girard F, Strausfield U, Fernandez A, Lamb NJC. Cyclin A is required for the onset of DNA replication in mammalian fibroblasts. Cell 1991;67:1169–79.
22. Walker DH, Maller JL. Role for cyclin A in the dependence of mitosis on completion of DNA replication. Nature 1991;354:314–7.
23. Devoto SH, Mudryj M, Pines J, Hunter T, Nevins JR. A cyclin A-protein kinase complex possesses sequence specific DNA binding activity: p33cdk2 is a component of the E2F-cyclin A complex. Cell 1992;68:167–76.
24. Ewen ME, Xing Y, Lawrence JB, Livingston DM. Molecular cloning, chromosomal mapping, and expression of the cDNA for p107, a retinoblastoma gene product-related protein. Cell 1991;66:1155–64.
25. Ewen ME, Faha B, Harlow E, Livingston DM. Interaction of p107 with cyclin A independent of complex formation with viral oncoproteins. Science 1992;255:85–7.
26. Mudryj M, Devoto SH, Hiebert SW, Hunter T, Pines J, Nevins JR. Cell cycle regulation of the E2F transcription factor involves an interaction with cyclin A. Cell 1991;65:1243–53.
27. Pagano M, Draetta G, Jansen-Durr P. Association of cdk2 kinase with the transcription factor E2F during S phase. Science 1992;255:1144–7.
28. Shirodkar S, Ewen M, Decaprio JA, Morgan J, Livingston DM, Chittenden T. The transcription factor E2F interacts with the retinoblastoma product and a p107-cyclin A complex in a cell cycle-regulated manner. Cell 1992;68:157–66.
29. Wang J, Chenivesse X, Henglein B, Brechot C. Hepatitis B virus integration in a cyclin A gene in hepatocellular carcinoma. Nature 1990;343:555–7.

30. Hadwiger JA, Wittenberg C, Richardson HE, Lopes MDB, Reed SI. A family of cyclin homologs that control the G1 phase in yeast. Proc Natl Acad Sci USA 1989;86:6255–9.
31. Wittenberg C, Sugimoto K, Reed SI. G1-specific cyclins of *S. cerevisiae*: cell cycle periodicity, regulation by mating pheromone, and association with the p34CDC28 protein kinase. Cell 1990;62:225–37.
32. Meyerson M, Enders GH, Wu C-L, et al. A family of human cdc2-related protein kinases. EMBO J 1992.
33. Koff A, Cross F, Fisher A, et al. Human cyclin E, a novel cyclin that interacts with two members of the CDC2 gene family. Cell 1991;66:1217–28.
34. Lew DJ, Dulic V, Reed SI. Isolation of three novel human cyclins by rescue of G1 cyclins (Cln) function in yeast. Cell 1991;66:1197–206.
35. Matsushime H, Roussel MF, Ashmun RA, Sherr CJ. Colony-stimulating factor 1 regulates novel cyclins during the G1 phase of the cell cycle. Cell 1991;65:701–13.
36. Xiong Y, Connolly T, Futcher B, Beach D. Human D-type cyclin. Cell 1991;65:691–9.
37. Draetta G, Luca F, Westendorf J, Brizuela L, Ruderman J, Beach D. cdc2 protein kinase is complexed with both cyclin A and B: evidence for proteolytic inactivation of MPF. Cell 1989;56:829–38.
38. Tsai L-H, Harlow E, Meyerson M. Isolation of the human cdk2 gene that encodes the cyclin A- and adenovirus E1A-associated p33 kinase. Nature 1991;353:174–7.
39. Elledge SJ, Richman R, Hall FL, Williams RT, Lodgson N, Harper JW. CDK2 encodes a 33-kDa cyclin A-associated protein kinase and is expressed before CDC2 in the cell cycle. Proc Natl Acad Sci USA 1992;89:2907–11.
40. Gould K, Nurse P. Tyrosine phosphorylation of the fission yeast cdc2+ protein kinase regulates entry into mitosis. Nature 1989;342:39–44.
41. Gould KL, Moreno S, Owen DJ, Sazer S, Nurse P. Phosphorylation at Thr167 is required for *Schizosaccharomyces pombe* p34cdc2 function. EMBO J 1991;10:3297–309.
42. Krek W, Nigg EA. Differential phosphorylation of vertebrate p34cdc2 kinase at the G1/S and G2/M transitions of the cell cycle: identification of major phosphorylation sites. EMBO J 1991;10:305–16.
43. Norbury C, Blow J, Nurse P. Regulatory phosphorylation of the p34cdc2 protein kinase in vertebrates. EMBO J 1991;10:3321–9.
44. Solomon MJ, Lee T, Kirschner MW. The role of phosphorylation in p34cdc2 activation: identification of an activating kinase. Mol Cell Biol 1992;3:13 27.
45. Dunphy W, Newport J. Fission yeast p13 blocks mitotic activation and tyrosine dephosphorylation of the *Xenopus* cdc2 protein kinase. Cell 1989;58:181–91.
46. Morla A, Draetta G, Beach D, Wang J. Reversible tyrosine phosphorylation of cdc2: dephosphorylation accompanies activation during entry into mitosis. Cell 1989;58:193–203.
47. Pines J, Hunter T. p34cdc2: the S and M kinase. New Biologist 1990;2:389–401.
48. Russell P, Nurse P. cdc25+ functions as an inducer in the mitotic control of fission yeast. Cell 1986;45:145–53.

49. Russell P, Nurse P. Negative regulation of mitosis by wee1+, a gene encoding a protein kinase homolog. Cell 1987;45:559–67.
50. Hanks S, Quinn A, Hunter T. The protein kinase family: conserved features and deduced phylogeny of the catalytic domains. Science 1988;241:42–52.
51. Lee MS, Ogg S, Xu M, et al. cdc25+ encodes a protein phosphatase that dephosphorylates p34cdc2. Mol Cell Biol 1992;3:73–84.
52. Parker LL, Atherton-Fessler S, Lee MS, et al. Cyclin promotes the tyrosine phosphorylation of p34cdc2 in a wee1+ dependent manner. EMBO J 1991;10:1255–63.
53. Parker LL, Atherton-Fessler S, Piwnica-Worms H. p107wee1 is a dual-specificity kinase that phosphorylates p34cdc2 on tyrosine 15. Proc Natl Acad Sci USA 1992;89:2917–21.
54. Featherstone C, Russell P. Fission yeast p107wee1 mitotic inhibitor is a tyrosine/serine kinase. Nature 1991;349:808–11.
55. Lindberg RA, Quinn AM, Hunter T. Dual-specificity protein kinases: will any hydroxyl do? TIBS 1992;17(March):114–9.
56. Dunphy WG, Kumagai A. The cdc25 protein contains an intrinsic phosphatase activity. Cell 1991;67:189–96.
57. Gautier J, Solomon MJ, Booher RN, Bazan JF, Kirschner MW. cdc25 is a specific tyrosine phosphatase that directly activates p3cdc2. Cell 1991;67:197–211.
58. Millar JBA, McGowan CH, Lenaers G, Jones R, Russell P. p80cdc25 mitotic inducer is the tyrosine phosphatase that activates p34cdc2 kinase in fission yeast. EMBO J 1991;10:4301–9.
59. Strausfeld U, Labbe JC, Fesquet D, et al. Dephosphorylation and activation of a p34cdc2/cyclin B complex in vitro by human CDC25 protein. Nature 1991;351:242–5.
60. Dailey D, Schieven GL, Lim MY, et al. Novel yeast protein kinase (YPK1 gene product) is a 40 Kd phosphotyrosyl protein associated with protein-tyrosine kinase activity. Mol Cell Biol 1990;10:6244–56.
61. Stern DF, Zheng P, Beidler DR, Zerillo C. Spk1, a new kinase from *S. cerevisiae*, phosphorylates proteins on serine, threonine and tyrosine. Mol Cell Biol 1991;11:987–1001.
62. Neigeborn L, Mitchekk AP. The yeast MCK1 gene encodes a protein kinase homolog that activates early meiotic expression. Genes Dev 1991;5:533–48.
63. Shero JH, Hieter P. A suppressor of a centromere DNA mutation encodes a putative protein kinase (MCK1). Genes Dev 1991;5:549–60.
64. Seger R, Ahn NG, Boulton TG, et al. Microtubule-associated protein 2 kinases ERK1 and ERK2 undergo autophosphorylation on both tyrosine and threonine residues: implications for their mechanism of activation. Proc Natl Acad Sci USA 1991;88:6142–6.
65. Wu J, Rossomando AJ, Her J-H, Del Vecchio R, Weber MJ, Sturgill TW. Autophosphorylation in vitro of recombinant 42-kilodalton mitogen-activated protein kinase on tyrosine. Proc Natl Acad Sci USA 1991;88:9508–12.
66. Crews CM, Alessandrini AA, Erikson RL. Mouse Erk-1 gene product is a serine/threonine protein kinase that has the potential to phosphorylate tyrosine. Proc Natl Acad Sci USA 1991;88:8845–9.

67. Howell BW, Afar DEH, Lew J, et al. STY, a tyrosine-phosphorylating enzyme with sequence homology to serine/threonine kinases. Mol Cell Biol 1991;11:568–72.
68. Ben-David Y, Letwin K, Tannock L, Bernstein A, Pawson T. A mammalian protein kinase with potential for serine/threonine and tyrosine phosphorylation is related to cell cycle regulators. EMBO J 1991;10:317–25.
69. Kaelin WG, Pallas DC, Decaprio JA, Kaye F, Livingston DM. Identification of cellular proteins that can interact specifically with the T/E1A-binding region of the retinoblastoma gene product. Cell 1991;64:521–32.
70. Moreno S, Nurse P. Clues to action of cdc25 protein. Science 1991;351:194.
71. Guan K, Broyles S, Dixon JE. A Tyr/Ser protein phosphatase encoded by vaccinia virus. Nature 1991;350:359–60.
72. Feilotter H, Nurse P, Young PG. Genetic and molecular analysis of cdr1/nim1 in *Schizosaccharomyces pombe*. Genetics 1991;127:309–18.
73. Russell P, Nurse P. The mitotic inducer nim+1 functions in a regulatory network of protein kinase homologs controlling the initiation of mitosis. Cell 1987;49:569–76.
74. Gould KL, Moreno S, Tonks N, Nurse P. Complementation of the mitotic activator, p80cdc25, by a human protein-tyrosine phosphatase. Science 1990; 250:1573–6.
75. Lundgren K, Walworth N, Booher R, Dembski M, Kirschner M, Beach D. mik1 and wee1 cooperate in the inhibitory tyrosine phosphorylation of cdc2. Cell 1991;64:1111–22.
76. Galaktionov K, Beach D. Specific activation of cdc25 tyrosine phosphatases by B-type cyclins: evidence for multiple roles of mitotic cyclins. Cell 1991; 67:1181–94.
77. Millar JBA, Blevitt J, Gerace L, Sadhu K, Featherstone C, Russell P. p55CDC25 is a nuclear protein required for the initiation of mitosis in human cells. Proc Natl Acad Sci USA 1991;88:10500–4.

# 6

# Hormonal Control of Cell-Cycle Checkpoints in Mammalian Oocytes

DAVID F. ALBERTINI, ANN E. ALLWORTH, AND
SUSAN M. MESSINGER

To coordinate ovum maturation with the initiation of embryonic development at fertilization, special modifications in female meiosis have occurred during the evolution of vertebrates. Fertilization in most vertebrates occurs between gametes that exist in distinctly different cell-cycle states. Sperm are postmeiotic, and oocytes are generally arrested at metaphase of meiosis 2 at the time of ovulation. While the completion of meiosis in oocytes is triggered by fertilization, several important checkpoints are imposed on meiotic cell-cycle progression throughout oogenesis to ensure that the events of meiotic M-phase are coordinated with follicular development and ovulation.

This chapter reviews M-phase of the meiotic cell cycle in mammalian oocytes with respect to a dualistic mode of regulation. First, evidence is considered indicating that the developmental acquisition and expression of meiotic competence—that is, the ability to initiate and execute M-phase—is a multistep process involving modulation of cell-cycle control gene products intrinsic to the oocyte. Second, information pertaining to the extrinsic hormonal modulation of cell-cycle control in oocytes is discussed relative to the presence of, and alterations in, cumulus cell–oocyte interactions. Given the limited amount of information available in both of these areas, it is hoped that the perspective provided in this chapter will facilitate the development of new experimental strategies for resolving the complex mechanisms that are involved in coordinating oogenesis, folliculogenesis, and ovulation.

## Meiotic M-Phase

### *When Is Prophase Prophase?*

Meiotic prophase in oocytes is classically viewed as a protracted state beginning with the formation of primary oocytes and ending shortly after the reinitiation of meiosis at ovulation. Unlike its somatic cell counterparts, however, the G2-like period of growth that would precede formal entry into mitotic prophase must overlap meiotic prophase during the growth phase of oogenesis if traditional semantics are accepted. There is no a priori reason to rigidly define the limits of meiotic prophase in view of currently accepted characteristics for the prophase state in somatic cells. For example, in somatic cells, several discrete and readily assayable cellular characteristics of mitotic prophase are widely recognized and include (i) loss of interphase *microtubules* (MTs), (ii) phosphorylation of centrosomes, (iii) chromatin condensation, (iv) nucleolar dissolution, (v) nuclear lamin disassembly, and (vi) dispersion of the Golgi complex (1). Directly or indirectly, the M-phase kinase that is activated at prophase onset in somatic cells is largely responsible for all of these structural alterations that antedate and are prerequisite for the execution of cell division. So, when is prophase prophase in a mammalian oocyte? A partial answer to this question rests in the analysis of the aforementioned cellular transformations during the process of oogenesis in mammals.

Studies on meiotic prophase in mouse oocytes indicate that formal entry into the M-phase of the cell cycle takes place at or around the time of meiotic competence acquisition. Supportive evidence for this idea is based on the observations that (i) germinal vesicle chromatin becomes condensed, especially around the nucleolus, at the time of antrum formation coincident with the loss of interphase MTs (2); (ii) the loss of interphase MTs occurs concomitant with the appearance of phosphorylated foci (3); and (iii) the functional expression of meiotic competence is associated with phosphorylation of centrosomes (4). While prognostic of entry into prophase, other signature features of the prophase transition are delayed in onset until *germinal vesicle breakdown* (GVBD) and include nucleolar dissolution, complete condensation of chromatin, and disassembly of nuclear lamins (1).

Thus, while some of the features of prophase entry appear during later stages of oogenesis, overt signs of this state do not appear until meiotic reinitiation just prior to GVBD. It appears that in the mouse, characteristics of prophase entry are partitioned throughout oogenesis in accordance with the conversion from a precompetent to competent meiotic state. It seems further that once competence is acquired, prophase is checked by extragametic components of the follicle that constitute the so-called meiotic arresting mechanism. Since prophase is a cell-cycle state regulated by the activation of the M-phase kinase, we next discuss what is known about the expression of this enzymatic activity in mammalian oocytes.

## M-Phase Kinase in Oocytes

Details concerning the biochemical composition and regulation of kinase activity of *maturation promoting factor* (MPF) have been reviewed (5 and see Piwnica-Worms, Chapter 5, this volume). Compared to the extensive literature on MPF in oocytes of lower vertebrates and invertebrates, there is relatively little known about MPF in mammalian oocytes. MPF was originally described as a cytoplasmic activity generated in maturing oocytes that upon transfer to immature GV-stage oocytes was capable of inducing meiotic maturation in a hormone-independent fashion. Therefore, cytoplasmic transfer of active MPF bypasses the hormone-dependent aspects of oocyte maturation. Cytoplasmic transfer and cell fusion experiments have shown that active MPF is generated during meiotic maturation in mouse oocytes (6, 7) and that this activity fluctuates, being maximal at metaphase of meiosis 1 and 2 and negligible at telophase of meiosis 1 (8).

Using histone *H1 kinase* (H1K) assays as an indicator of MPF activity, similar stage-specific fluctuations have been noted in both pig (9) and mouse oocytes (8), and in the latter studies, it was shown additionally that the appearance of H1K activity is associated with dephosphorylation of Tyr-15 on the $p34^{cdc2}$ catalytic subunit. Interestingly, this group also demonstrated that *isobutylmethylxanthine* (IBMX), a phosphodiesterase inhibitor known to maintain mouse oocytes in meiotic arrest by elevating intraoocytic cAMP, causes $p34^{cdc2}$ Tyr-15 phosphorylation; this modification would be expected to prevent activation of the M-phase kinase. The significance of this finding with respect to the regulation of meiosis is best appreciated by consideration of two additional aspects of oocyte and follicle metabolism that have been studied in rodents.

First, it has long been recognized that meiotic resumption in the mouse proceeds to prometaphase in the presence of inhibitors of protein synthesis (10). Moreover, when oocytes are arrested in IBMX in the presence of protein synthesis inhibitors, they lose the ability to resume meiosis in a protein synthesis-independent fashion (11). Collectively, these observations indicate that meiotically competent mouse oocytes contain sufficient stores of MPF or factors modulating its activation to direct the early events of maturation without new protein synthesis, even in the absence of cumulus cells. Thus, conditions established during oogenesis provide a mechanism for meiotic cell-cycle control that is intrinsic to the oocyte.

Second, it is now appreciated that hormone-mediated responses in cumulus cells modulate the expression of meiotic competence. In vitro and in vivo evidence supportive of this idea is that (i) factors such as cAMP are believed to originate in cumulus cells and inhibit maturation in vivo, (ii) hormonal stimulation of cumulus-enclosed oocytes is needed for the completion of maturation, and (iii) under culture conditions that maintain meiotic arrest, factors such as EGF or FSH have been shown to positively induce meiotic resumption (12). Given the fact that both stimulatory and inhibitory mechanisms can be invoked to explain meiotic competence through cumulus cell-oocyte interactions, it is imperative that the modes of interaction between these two cell types be rigorously defined.

## Cumulus Cell-Oocyte Interactions

Various aspects of meiotic M-phase in oocytes are thought to be regulated by germ cell interaction with surrounding cumulus cells. With respect to prophase, it is likely that entry into, maintenance of, and release from the prophase-arrested state involve different forms of information transfer during oogenesis and folliculogenesis. At least two types of interactions underlie somatic cell-to-gamete information transfer. The first mode of interaction is thought to be mediated by *gap junctions*, intercellular specializations of apposed plasma membranes that permit the direct passage of low molecular weight substances. Gap junctions are ubiquitous at the interface between cumulus cells and oocytes in many mammalian species (13, 14), and ionic coupling and metabolic cooperation have been shown to occur in some species (14, 15).

The simplest form of gap junction-mediated cell-cycle regulation in oocytes could involve transfer of second messengers—such as cyclic nucleotides, ions, or lipids ($IP_3$)—from cumulus cells to the ooplasm, where direct inhibitory or stimulatory actions of these agents would either directly or indirectly modulate MPF activity. While no direct data are available to support such a mechanism in mammals, hormone-induced mobilization of calcium in follicle cells and its transfer to oocytes in amphibians have recently been documented (16). This study also raises the possibility that acute hormone responses in cumulus cells may modulate gating of the connexon subunits that comprise gap junctions. Further work will be required to improve our understanding of how gap junction-mediated interactions participate in the control of meiotic cell-cycle progression in the mammalian ovarian follicle.

Intercellular junctions other than gap junctions are also known to exist at juxtaposed cumulus cell-oocyte plasma membranes. These junctions exhibit fine structural characteristics of adhesive connections, such as macula adherens (13), and as such, are likely to involve extracellular calcium and *cell adhesion molecules* (CAMs) to ensure their physical integrity. While very little is known about their distribution, composition, or function in the mammalian cumulus-oocyte complex, certain features of the organization of adhesive junctions make them particularly appealing for future study.

For example, adhesive junctions provide stable contact zones at the oolemma that, by virtue of their local sites of binding, could directly influence receptor activity or fluidity in the oocyte plasma membrane. In addition, extensive zones of adhesion at the ends of transzonal processes would effectively constitute domains of membrane at which exocytotic events could take place. As in the neuromuscular junction, it seems plausible that specialized zones of adhesion between oocytes and cumulus cells may be required to ensure vectorial transport and exocytosis of cumulus cell products into the perivitelline space. There may be merit in adopting this perspective since there is mounting evidence to suggest that gamete or cumulus cell secretions may modulate cumulus-oocyte complex physiology through paracrine routes of stimulation (17, 18). Moreover, we have recently demonstrated that in vitro cumulus expansion of bovine cumulus-oocyte complexes involves a dramatic cytoskeletal transformation of the cumulus cells (unpublished observations).

It has been known for many years that cumulus cells of most mammalian species extend slender cytoplasmic processes that traverse the zona pellucida to make junctional contact with the oolemma (13, 14). Indeed, in the rodent it has been hypothesized that the disruption of cumulus cell processes around the time of GVBD effectively removes a meiotic inhibitory signal imposed by cumulus cell-generated cAMP. In the cow, while the frequency of gap junctions also decreases around the time of GVBD (19), a different mode of cumulus cell communication may be established. At the onset of maturation, transzonal cumulus cell processes are short, slender, and microfilament rich; however, over the course of maturation, these are replaced by long, thick, microtubule-rich cumulus cell processes. While the functional significance of these processes has not been established, it is tempting to speculate that they provide bidirectional signal transduction pathways between the cumulus cells and the oocyte. Unlike rodents, oocytes from domestic species cannot proceed through meoisis in the absence of protein synthesis (5). Therefore, it is possible that extragametic input may elicit signals required for meiotic progression. The extent to which hormones elicit synthesis, transport, and local release of paracrine-acting factors in cumulus cells is not presently known, but stands as an area for active investigation in the future.

## Summary

Meiotic cell-cycle progression during oogenesis in mammals is hormonally regulated as a result of the ability of cells within the cumulus-oocyte complex to function as a syncytium. Following this synthesis during oogenesis, the cell-cycle control molecules required for meiotic maturation are modulated by inputs received from somatic cumulus cells. It appears that at least two modes of interactions between cumulus cells and oocytes regulate meiotic progression. Direct inputs are mediated by gap junctions, whereas adhesive junctions are proposed to mediate both cell-contact-dependent and secretory events that collectively coordinate follicular development with gametogenesis.

*Acknowledgment.* This work was supported by NIH Grant HD-20068.

## References

1. Albertini DF, Mattson B, Messinger SM, Wickramasinghe D, Plancha CE. Nuclear and cytoplasmic changes during oocyte maturation. In: Bavister BD, ed. Preimplantation embryo development. New York: Springer-Verlag, 1993.
2. Mattson BA, Albertini DF. Oogenesis: chromatin and microtubule dynamics during meiotic prophase. Mol Reprod Dev 1990;25:374–83.
3. Wickramasinghe D, Ebert KM, Albertini DF. Meiotic competence acquisition is associated with the appearance of M-phase characteristics in growing mouse oocytes. Dev Biol 1991;143:162–72.
4. Wickramasinghe D, Albertini DF. Centrosome phosphorylation and the developmental expression of meiotic competence in mouse oocytes. Dev Biol 1992;152:62–74.
5. Albertini DF. Regulation of meiotic maturation in the mammalian oocyte: interplay between exogenous cues and the microtubule cytoskeleton. Bioessays 1992;14:97–103.
6. Balakier H. Induction of maturation in small oocytes from sexually immature mice by fusion with meiotic and mitotic cells. Exp Cell Res 1977;112:137–41.
7. Sorensen RA, Cyert MS, Pedersen RA. Active maturation-promoting factor is present in mature mouse oocytes. J Cell Biol 1985;100:1637–40.
8. Choi T, Aoki F, Mori M, Yamashita M, Nagahama Y, Kohmoto K. Activation of p34/cdc2 protein kinase in meiotic and mitotic cycles of mouse oocytes and embryos. Development 1991;113(3):789–96.
9. Naito K, Daen FP, Toyoda Y. Comparison of histone H1 kinase activity during meiotic maturation between two types of porcine oocytes matured in different media in vitro. Biol Reprod 1992;47:43–7.
10. Schultz RM, Wassarman PM. Biochemical studies of mammalian oogenesis: protein synthesis during oocyte growth and meiotic maturation in the mouse. J Cell Sci 1977;24:167–94.
11. Downs SM. Protein synthesis inhibitors prevent both spontaneous and hormone-dependent maturation of isolated mouse oocytes. Mol Reprod Dev 1990;27:235–43.
12. Buccione R, Schroeder AC, Eppig JJ. Interactions between somatic cells and germ cells throughout mammalian oogenesis. Biol Reprod 1990;43:543–7.
13. Anderson E, Albertini DF. Gap junctions between the oocyte and companion follicle cells in the mammalian ovary. J Cell Biol 1976;71:680–6.
14. Gilula NB, Epstein ML, Beers WH. Cell-to-cell communication and ovulation: a study of the cumulus-oocyte complex. J Cell Biol 1978;78:58–75.

15. Phillips DM, Dekel N. Maturation of the rat cumulus-oocyte complex: structure and function. Mol Reprod Dev 1991;28:297–306.
16. Sandberg K, Bor K, Ji H, Marwick A, Millan MA, Catt KJ. Angiotensin II-induced calcium mobilization in oocytes by signal transfer through gap junctions. Science 1990;249:298–301.
17. Buccione R, Vanderhyden BC, Caron PJ, Eppig JJ. FSH-induced expansion of the mouse cumulus oophorus in vitro is dependent upon a specific factor(s) secreted by the oocyte. Dev Biol 1990;138:16–25.
18. Salustri A, Yanagishita M, Hascall VC. Mouse oocytes regulate hyaluronic acid synthesis and mucification by FSH-stimulated cumulus cells. Dev Biol 1990;138:26–32.
19. Hyttel P. Bovine cumulus-oocyte disconnection in vitro. Anat Embryol 1987;176:41–4.

# Part II

# Gonadotropin Receptor and Control Mechanisms

# 7
# Structure and Regulation of the LH Receptor Gene and Its Transcripts

TAE H. JI, YONG BUM KOO, AND INHAE JI

Expression of the LH receptor is tightly regulated by hormones and is dependent on development of the ovary and differentiation of ovarian cells (1, 2). The recent cloning of LH receptor cDNAs (3, 4) has made it possible to find a number of transcripts whose sizes vary from 7.8 kb to 1.2 kb as well as the genomic structure (5–11). We have isolated overlapping Cosmid clones spanning over 90 kb from 23 kb upstream of the translation start site of the rat LH receptor gene to 13 kb downstream of the stop codon (Fig. 7.1). The rat LH receptor gene spans over 70 kb. The coding region is more than 60 kb and consists of 11 exons and 10 introns (12, 13). The first 10 exons encode the extracellular N-terminal half of the receptor, while exon 11 encodes the C-terminal half of the receptor that includes the 7 transmembrane helices. Restriction maps and gene dose analyses of exons 1 and 11 demonstrate that a single-copy gene encodes the LH receptor (19). The gene does not have a TATA box and may utilize an initiator(s) in place of a TATA box for transcription.

## Transcription Start Sites

Transcription start sites are important not only for establishing the first nucleotide of transcripts, but also as initiators to control a transcriptional regulatory element, particularly in TATA-less genes, such as the LH receptor gene (14, 15). Furthermore, the use of alternate initiators in a gene with multiple transcription start sites correlates with the promoter strength (14). In addition, they define the upstream translational regulatory region of mRNAs (16).

It has been reported that there are two groups of multiple transcription start sites in the rat LH receptor gene: proximal and upstream start sites (13). Our results are not entirely consistent with the report. Several

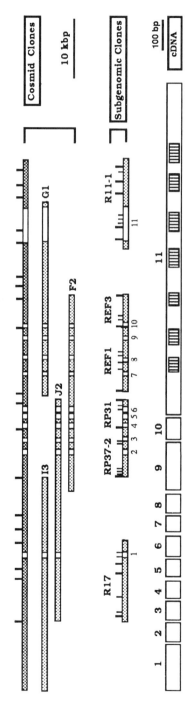

FIGURE 7.1. Organization of the rat LH receptor gene. Four overlapping Cosmid clones (I3, J2, F2, and G1) span over 90 kb from 23 kb upstream of the translation start site to 13 kb downstream of the stop codon. These clones cover 6 nonoverlapping subgenomic clones (R17, RP37-2, RP31, REF1, REF3, and R11-1) that include all 11 exons found in the coding sequence. R17, REF1, and R11-1 are lGEM 11 clones, and the others are pGEM 11Zf+ clones. The thick vertical lines are *Eco*RI sites, and the thin lines are *Sac*I sites. The clear boxes indicate the locations of exons. The lined boxes within exon 11 represent transmembrane domains. The first 10 exons encode the N-terminal half of the molecule, while exon 11 encodes the C-terminal half of the molecule, which includes all 7 putative transmembrane domains and the entire C-terminal cytoplasmic domain.

# 7. Structure and Regulation of the LH Receptor Gene and Its Transcripts 91

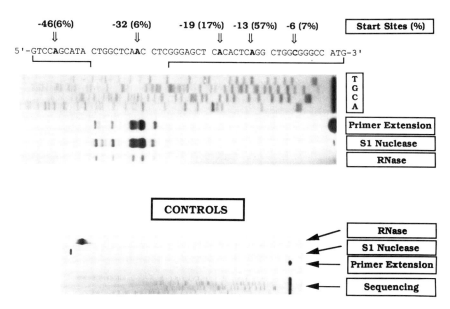

FIGURE 7.2. Determination of transcription start sites. Primer extension, S1 nuclease protection, and RNAse protection were carried out with primer and cRNA probes shown in controls.

independent methods were employed in our study, including S1 nuclease protection, RNAse protection, primer extension, cloning and sequencing, and Northern hybridization. Each of these methods has strengths and weaknesses. Primer extension and S1 nuclease protection produce clean results, but can produce artificial sites due to the potential inaccessibility of polymerase and S1 nuclease. On the other hand, RNAse can thoroughly digest samples while producing dirty results.

In primer extension, a number of different primers were used starting at positions of $-2036$, $-1304$, $-1957$, $-694$, $-235$, $-48$, and $+152$. This approach was to ensure the full coverage of the proximal and distant upstream regions that might be interrupted by presumptive introns. As shown in Figure 7.2, five common conspicuous transcription start sites were identified in the proximal region by primer extension, S1 nuclease protection, and RNA protection. They are at positions of $-46$, $-32$, $-19$, $-13$, and $-6$, with relative band intensities of 6%, 6%, 17%, 57%, and 7%, respectively. The $-13$ site is the strongest, followed by the $-19$ site. Since the determination of start sites by these methods can be misleading, we followed a more definitive approach to cloning and sequencing. Three clones showed the start sites at positions of $-46$, $-19$, and $-13$. Upstream start sites, however, were not detected, although some weak bands appeared in our preliminary experiments that turned out to be false in high-stringency tests.

To further verify our results, mRNAs isolated from superovulated rat ovaries were hybridized with cRNA probes of the N-terminal coding region or an upstream genomic cRNA probe spanning from −189 to −1055. From our experience, RNA with a >50 base sequence homology should be detected by this approach. However, no band was detected, consistent with our results in Figure 7.2. To further examine these results, PCR products of mRNAs were analyzed. There was one band of 120 bp that represents mRNAs with the proximal start sites. These results are in accord with our observation that a hyperactive regulatory region is present in the region between −187 to −25 and a functional *activating protein 2 responsive element* (AP2E) exists in the region between −60 and −51.

An examination of the upstream sequence indicates that there is no sequence that is similar to the consensus CCAAT motif and TATA element within 700 bp upstream of the transcription start sites (Fig. 7.2). This result, taken together with the presence of multiple proximal start sites, indicates a promoter without the CCAAT and TATA boxes.

## Regulatory Region

To define the regulatory region of the LH receptor gene, upstream gene fragments were inserted in front of the luciferase coding sequence in a eukaryotic expression vector. These fragments are −6.5 kb to −25 b, −2074 to −25, −1376 to −25, −187 to −25, −2074 to +30, and −2074 to +150. These constructs were transfected into *murine Leydig tumor cells* (MLTC) that constitutively express the LH receptor. Luciferase activity was highest with the construct containing the sequence from −187 to −25, while the −6.5 kb to −25 b construct showed the lowest activity. Promoterless vector did not show any noticeable activity. The results indicate that these DNA sequences have promoter activities. The −187 to −25 sequence is hyperactive, whereas there are strong repressor sequences in the region from −6.5 kb to −25 b. Downstream extension of the DNA fragments up to +150 b resulted in a slight reduction of the activity, indicating that the downstream sequence has a weak negative activity. To characterize the hyperactive −187 to −25 region, the DNA fragment was inserted in the reverse orientation into the vector. A 50% reduction in luciferase activity was observed, indicating that the −187 to −25 sequence functions in both orientations, but less effectively in the reverse orientation.

Since the LH receptor gene is induced by cAMP (17, 18), we looked for *cAMP responsive elements* (CRE) upstream of the transcription start sites. No consensus CRE (19, 20) was found in this region, but there was an AP2E. This sequence is responsive to both cAMP and kinase C and appears to be tissue specific and independent of the position, unlike the ubiquitous consensus CRE upstream of the transcription start sites (21).

7. Structure and Regulation of the LH Receptor Gene and Its Transcripts    93

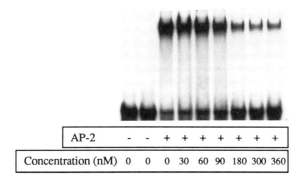

FIGURE 7.3. Gel mobility shift. End-labeled double-strand AP2E was incubated with AP2 extracts in the presence of increasing concentrations of cold double-strand AP2E. The resulting mixture was electrophoresed on a gel.

We have constructed a vector with the AP2E sequence. It showed a weak promoter activity. To test that the AP2E in the LH receptor gene is active, the constructs were cotransfected with an expression vector containing AP2. Coexpression resulted in decreases of luciferase activity when the constructs containing the sequences −2074 to +30 and −2074 to +150 were used. These results indicate that the LH receptor gene sequences are affected by the presence of AP2 and that the AP2E may be active. Therefore, the weak repressor activity observed with the downstream sequences appears to be amplified in the presence of expressed AP2.

However, the gene sequences lacking the downstream sequence remained as active as before. On the other hand, the reversed −25 to −187 sequence, which has 50% of the activity of the sequence with the right orientation, recovered the full activity when the construct was cotransfected with the AP2 construct. This result clearly demonstrates the involvement of AP2 in the luciferase expression. Furthermore, it suggests that the gene expression is dependent on the concentration of AP2 and that the regulatory protein is involved in gene expression both positively and negatively.

All these results, however, fail to demonstrate that the AP2E of the LH receptor interact with AP2. It is known that not only core regulatory DNA sequences but also their flanking sequences are important for binding to proteins. Therefore, it is necessary to test whether or not the AP2E in the LH receptor gene indeed binds AP2. To examine their binding, double-strand AP2E sequence was end labeled, incubated with AP2, and electrophoresed. The result shows both their binding and that the binding can be blocked by unlabeled double-strand AP2E (Fig. 7.3). The Kd value was in the range of nM. Furthermore, the binding appears to be specific, as single-strand AP2Es failed to block the binding. Apparently, AP2 recognizes double-strand DNA sequence, unlike other proteins that are capable of binding both single- and double-strand DNAs.

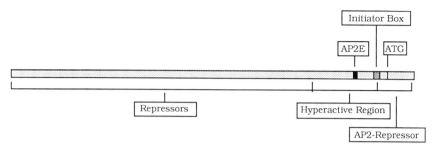

FIGURE 7.4. Regulatory region of the LH receptor gene.

Figure 7.4 summarizes the regulatory region. There are multiple alternate transcription start sites between the −46 and −6 positions. They may comprise initiators. In the immediate upstream of the initiator box is the hyperactive region, including a functional AP2E. This hyperactive region is flanked by repressor sequences. Strong repressor activities are found in the distant upstream, while weak AP2-dependent repressor activity is located in the proximal downstream.

## LH Receptor mRNA

Northern analyses of LH receptor messages isolated from pseudopregnant rat ovaries and rat testes have shown conspicuous signals at the positions of 7.8, 7, 4.2, 2.5, 1.8, and 1.25 kb (5–11). The 1.8 and 1.25 kb messages, which are expected to encode truncated receptors as the full coding sequence is nearly 2 kb, are expressed transcriptionally and developmentally in rat ovaries and testes, respectively (5, 6). Also, transcripts smaller than 1.25 kb appear to be present in fetal and neonatal rat ovaries up to 7 days postpartum (22). Despite the developmental regulation of this selective expression of truncated LH receptor messages, their structures, as well as the structures of various other sizes of LH receptor transcripts, are not well defined. The understanding of the functions of these messages necessitates the characterization of their structures. Truncated messages may competitively inhibit translation simply by occupying the translation machinery and encode truncated receptors that could inhibit the processing and activity of the normal receptor.

To identify variant LH receptor transcripts, mRNAs were isolated and used for PCR with a number of 3′ primers starting at positions of +176, +895, +1723, +2753, and +3745. A variety of PCR products of discrete sizes were produced, cloned, and sequenced. The results are summarized in Figure 7.5. Clone I-3 continued from exon 3 into intron 3 and was polyadenylated in intron 3. Likewise, clones I-4 and I-10 were polyadenylated in intron 4 and intron 10, respectively. Interestingly, the open reading frame of these clones terminates with a termination codon 4 bases

7. Structure and Regulation of the LH Receptor Gene and Its Transcripts 95

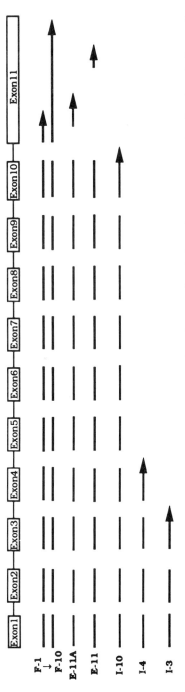

FIGURE 7.5. Alternately spliced LH receptor mRNAs and their polyadenylation sites. The arrowhead points indicate the positions of polyadenylation sites.

TABLE 7.1. [$^{125}$I]hCG binding and intracellular cAMP induction. The 293 cells were transfected with various constructs. Intact transfected cells, Triton X-100 extracts of the cells, and cell culture supernatants were assayed for [$^{125}$I]hCG binding and intracellular cAMP synthesis.

| LH receptor | Source | Kd (nM) | EC$_{50}$ for cAMP (nM) |
|---|---|---|---|
| Wild-type | Intact cells | 0.30 | 0.05 |
| | TX-100 extract | 0.32 | — |
| | Supernatant | ND | — |
| E-11A | Intact cells | ND | ND |
| | TX-100 extract | 0.29 | — |
| | Supernatant | ND | — |
| I-10 | Intact cells | ND | ND |
| | TX-100 extract | 0.30 | — |
| | Supernatant | ND | — |
| I-3 | Intact cells | ND | ND |
| | TX-100 extract | 24.80 | — |
| | Supernatant | ND | — |
| I-4 | Intact cells | ND | ND |
| | TX-100 extract | 27.50 | — |
| | Supernatant | ND | — |

downstream of the exon-intron junctions. Furthermore, the penultimate terminal codons in all three cases are CTG to encode leucine. Therefore, these clones are expected to yield soluble N-terminal peptides. Exon 10 of clones E-11 and E-11A was spliced to bases in the middle of exon 11, instead of the normal splicing to the beginning of exon 11. The reading frame of both clones was switched and ended with a termination codon not too far downstream. These clones are also expected to produce soluble forms of the LH receptor. Clones F-1 to F-4 have the full-length coding sequence with different polyadenylation sites.

In some of the truncated receptor clones, the polyadenylation sites are preceded by TTTTTAT, which is a consensus sequence for the activation of cytoplasmic polyadenylation. It is of interest to know whether they are involved in the regulation of cytoplasmic polyadenylation and, therefore, the regulation of LH receptor mRNAs themselves.

To determine the functions of the cDNAs of truncated LH receptors, binding of [$^{125}$I]hCG was performed with transfected 293 cells, cells solubilized in Triton X-100, and culture supernatants. In addition, intracellular cAMP synthesis induced by hCG was also determined with intact transfected cells. As shown in Table 7.1, neither the intact 293 cells that were transfected with clones I-3, I-4, I-10, and E-11A nor their culture supernatants showed cAMP induction. In contrast, the cells transfected with the wild-type LH receptor construct recognized [$^{125}$I]hCG with Kd values of 0.30–0.32 nM. In addition, these cells responded to

# 7. Structure and Regulation of the LH Receptor Gene and Its Transcripts

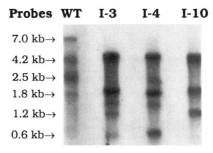

FIGURE 7.6. Northern hybridization of LH receptor mRNA. The mRNAs were isolated from superovulated rat ovaries, electrophoresed on agarose gel, and hybridized with a probe of the N-terminal coding region of the LH receptor (WT), intron 3 probe (I-3), intron 4 probe (I-4), or intron 10 probe (I-10).

hCG to produce cAMP with an $EC_{50}$ value of 0.05 nM. When transfected cells were solubilized in Triton X-100, the extracts of the cells transfected with clones I-3, I-4, I-10, and E-11A showed [$^{125}$I]hCG binding with Kd values of 24.8, 27.5, 0.30, and 0.29 nM, respectively.

These results indicate several important points. The short I-3 and I-4 mRNAs are translatable and, therefore, are capable of competing with full-length LH receptor mRNAs for translation. Furthermore, the peptides that are encoded by these alternately spliced mRNAs are capable of binding the hormone with considerable affinities, therefore indicating that there is at least one hormone contact point in the receptor peptide encoded by exons 1–3. This conclusion is consistent with the existence of multiple hormone contact points in the receptor (23–25) and the ability of the receptor's N-terminal half to bind the hormone (23, 26, 27).

To examine natural forms of LH receptor mRNAs containing introns, LH receptor mRNAs were hybridized with cRNA probes specific for introns 3, 4, and 10. As shown in Figure 7.6, introns 3 and 4 were found in the mRNAs of 4.2-, 1.8-, 1.2-, and 0.6-kb bands, whereas the probe for the N-terminal half of the LH receptor identified 7.0-, 4.2-, 2.5-, and 1.8-kb bands. The results clearly demonstrate the existence of variant mRNA containing the introns and their various sizes. Apparently, 7.0-, and 2.5-kb mRNAs do not have introns 3, 4, and 10. Furthermore, the results underscore the significant heterogeneity of each LH receptor mRNA band.

We failed, however, to isolate clones of exon 1 and exons 1–2. Whether this failure means the absence of corresponding mRNAs with distinct biological roles is yet to be determined and may have some significant implications. For example, if exon 1 and exons 1–2 mRNAs are indeed absent, these mRNAs, which are shorter than mRNAs of exons 1–3 and 1–4, may not be transcribed at all, suggesting the existence of intriguing transcriptional regulatory mechanisms for selective expression. Furthermore, it has added interest for the potential functions of exons 1–3 and 1–4 mRNAs and their peptide products.

We have identified two short mRNAs of LH receptor exons 1-3 and exons 1-4. It is of interest to compare these mRNAs with those expressed during the early developmental stages of the fetal and neonatal rat ovaries (22). If they are indentical, our results would indicate that the exon 1-3 and 1-4 mRNAs are present as predominant species during the early developmental stage, while they are extremely minor species in the mature stage of rat ovaries. It is important to determine whether such differential expression is due to either different transcription rates or different stabilities.

*Acknowledgment.* This work was supported by Grant AG-10559 from the National Institutes of Health.

## References

1. Richards JS. Maturation of ovarian follicles: actions and interactions of pituitary and ovarian hormones on follicular development. Physiol Rev 1980; 60:51-89.
2. Adashi EY, Hsueh AJW. Hormonal induction of receptors during ovarian granulosa cell differentiation. Receptors 1984;1:587-626.
3. McFarland KC, Sprengel R, Phillips HS, et al. Lutropin-choriogonadotropin receptor: an unusal member of the G protein-coupled receptor family. Science 1989;245:525-8.
4. Loosfelt H, Misrahi M, Atger M, et al. Cloning and sequencing of porcine LH-hCG receptor cDNA: variant lacking transmembrane domain. Science 1989;245:525-8.
5. LaPolt PS, Jia X-C, Sincich C, Hsueh AJW. Ligand-induced down-regulation of testicular and ovarian luteinizing hormone (LH) receptor is preceded by tissue-specific inhibition of alternatively processed LH transcripts. Mol Endocrinol 1991;5:397-403.
6. Vihko KK, Nishimori K, LaPolt PS. LH and FSH receptor mRNA in the rat testis: developmental regulation of mutiple transcripts during postnatal life. Biol Reprod 1991;44(suppl 1):476.
7. Frazier AL, Robbins LS, Stork PJ, Sprengel R, Segaloff DL, Cone RD. Isolation of TSH and LH/CG receptor cDNAs from human thyroid: regulation by tissue specific splicing. Mol Endocrinol 1990;4:1264-76.
8. Bernard MP, Myers RV, Moyle WR. Cloning of rat lutropin (LH) receptor analogs lacking the soybean lectin domain. Mol Cell Endocrinol 1990;71: R19-23.
9. Tsai-Morris CH, Buczko E, Wang W, Dufau ML. Intronic nature of the rat luteinizing hormone receptor gene defines a soluble receptor subspecies with hormone binding activity. J Biol Chem 1990;265:19385-8.
10. LaPolt PS, Oikawa M, Jia X-C, Dargan C, Hsueh AJW. Gonadotropin-induced up- and down-regulation of rat ovarian LH receptor message levels during follicular growth, ovulation and luteinization. Endocrinology 1990; 126:3277-9.

11. Wang H, Ascoli M, Seagaloff DL. Multiple luteinizing hormone/chorionic gonadotropin receptor messenger ribonucleic acid transcripts. Endocrinology 1991;129:133–8.
12. Koo YB, Ji I, Slaughter RG, Ji TH. Structure of the luteinizing hormone receptor gene and multiple exons of the coding sequence. Endocrinology 1991;128:2297–308.
13. Tsai-Morris CH, Buczko E, Wang W, Xie X-Z, Dufau ML. Structural organization of the rat luteinizing hormone (LH) receptor gene. J Biol Chem 1991;266:11355–9.
14. Smale ST, Baltimore D. The "initiator" as a transcription control element. Cell 1989;57:103–13.
15. O'Shea-Greenfield, Smale ST. Roles of TATA and initiator elements in determining the start site location and direction of RNA polymerase II transcription. J Biol Chem 1992;267:1391–402.
16. Theil EC. Regulation of ferritin and transferrin receptor mRNAs. J Biol Chem 1990;265:4771–4.
17. LaPolt PS, Oikawa M, Jia X-C, Dargan C, Hsueh AJW. Gonadotropin-induced up- and down-regulation of rat LH receptor message levels during follicular growth, ovulation and luteinization. Endocrinology 1990;126:3277–9.
18. Segaloff DL, Wang H, Richards JS. Hormone-specific regulation of LH/CG receptor mRNA expression in rat ovarian follicles and corpora lutea. Proc 72nd annu meet Endocr Soc. Atlanta, 1990:290.
19. Silver BJ, Bokar JA, Virgin JB, Vallen EA, Milsted A, Nilson JH. Cyclic AMP regulation of the human glycoprotein hormone alpha-subunit gene is mediated by an 18-base-pair element. Proc Natl Acad Sci USA 1987;84:2198–202.
20. Roesler WJ, Vandenbark GR, Hansen RW. Cyclic AMP and the induction of eukaryotic gene transcription. J Biol Chem 1988;263:9063–6.
21. Imagawa M, Chiu R, Karin M. Transcriptional factor AP-2 mediates induction by two different signal-transduction pathways: protein kinase C and cAMP. Cell 1987;51:251–60.
22. Sokka T, Hamalainen T, Huhtaniemi I. Functional LH receptor appears in the neonatal rat ovary after changes in the alternative splicing pattern of the LH receptor mRNA. Endocrinology 1992;130:1738–40.
23. Ji I, Ji TH. Exons 1–10 of the rat LH receptor encode a high affinity hormone binding site and exon 11 encodes G-protein modulation and a potential second hormone binding site. Endocrinology 1991;128:2648–50.
24. Ji I, Ji TH. Both α and β subunits of human choriogonadotropin photoaffinity label the hormone receptor. Proc Natl Acad Sci 1981;78:5465–9.
25. Ryan RJ, Charlesworth MC, McCormick DJ, Milius RP, Keutmann HT. The glycoprotein hormones: recent studies of structure-function relationships. FASEB J 1988;2:2661–9.
26. Tsai-Morris CH, Buczko E, Wang W, Dufau ML. Intronic nature of the rat luteinizing hormone receptor gene defines a soluble receptor subspecies with hormone binding activity. J Biol Chem 1990;265:19385–8.
27. Xie YB, Wang H, Segaloff DL. Extracellular domain of lutropin/choriogonadotropin receptor expressed in transfected cells binds choriogonadotropin with high affinity. J Biol Chem 1990;265:21411–4.

# 8
# Regulation of Expression of the FSH Receptor

MICHAEL D. GRISWOLD AND LESLIE L. HECKERT

*Follicle stimulating hormone* (follitropin [FSH]) is a pituitary glycoprotein hormone that is essential for normal reproduction in both male and female mammals. Sertoli cells and granulosa cells are the target cells for the action of FSH in the testes and ovaries, respectively. The function of the Sertoli cells includes the physical and biochemical support for germ cell development into spermatozoa. Sertoli cells create an environment where germ cells are provided with metabolites, nutrients, and physical support. Granulosa cells have similar overall functions in the ovary; that is, they play a role in the overall support of the ovum and the development of the follicle (reviewed in 1–3). According to this scenario, FSH indirectly influences spermatogenesis and oogenesis by exerting influences on the corresponding somatic cells (1, 2, 4–7). The primary action of FSH is mediated by increased concentrations of intracellular cAMP (8, 9). There is also evidence that FSH can alter intracellular calcium levels through mechanisms that are independent of both the protein kinase C pathway and the adenylate cyclase activity (10, 11).

## Sertoli and Granulosa Cells

The granulosa cells of the ovary and the Sertoli cells of the testis share a number of similarities that have been noted previously (12). Both cell types are necessary for the development and survival of the germ cells prior to ovulation or spermatogenesis. Although the determination of the embryological origin of these cells has been difficult, it has been postulated that Sertoli cells and granulosa cells originate from a common precursor cell (12). Immature and mature granulosa and Sertoli cells have some similar biochemical properties, including the synthesis of some of the same proteins, such as plasminogen activator and inhibin. Both granulosa cells and immature Sertoli cells are capable of synthesizing estrogens from an exogenous source of androgens (12). The major similarity between the two cell types, however, is that both cells are target cells for the action of FSH, and they are the only cell types that are thought to express the FSH receptor. It is possible that the transcriptional machinery that regulates the expression of the FSH receptor is similar in both granulosa cells and Sertoli cells.

In addition to the obvious similarities between the two gonadal somatic cell types, there are also some important differences. The Sertoli cells are very large cells ($30 \times 80\,\mu m$), each of which physically and biochemically supports many germ cells (12–15). Tight junctional complexes between adjacent Sertoli cells confine the region of cellular interaction with FSH to the 5% of the plasma membrane that is basal to these junctional complexes (13, 16). While FSH is a mitogen to prepubertal Sertoli cells, the adult population of Sertoli cells is fixed early in development (17, 18). Granulosa cells, on the other hand, are not as large as Sertoli cells, and an abundant population of granulosa cells provides biochemical support to a single large germ cell. A junctional complex equivalent to that between Sertoli cells does not form between adjacent granulosa cells, and FSH can interact with a large fraction of the cellular membrane (1). FSH is a mitogen to granulosa cells throughout follicular development (7). In addition, the synthesis of LH receptors triggered by the action of FSH is unique to granulosa cells (7).

## FSH Receptor

The *follicle stimulating hormone receptor* (FSH-R), like the receptors for LH/CG and TSH, is a member of a family of receptors that act via interactions with G-proteins (19–22). This receptor family includes the adrenergic, muscarinic cholinergic, dopamine, and substance K receptors, as well as the visual pigment rhodopsin and the putative G-21 protein (19–26). All these receptors traverse the plasma membrane with 7 α-helices oriented with an extracellular amino terminus and an intracellular carboxy terminus (26, 27). The primary amino acid sequence in the membrane-spanning regions is highly conserved within members of this family (21, 26). The amino acid sequences deduced from the cloned cDNA for many receptors in this family reveal major differences between the distinct receptors in the size of the extracellular domain (19, 20, 22, 24–26, 28–31). In general, the glycoprotein hormone receptors have very large, extensive, amino terminal domains, while all others in this family have short amino terminal domains. The cDNA for FSH-R was shown to encode a 675-amino acid, 75-kd protein with a 348-amino acid external domain (22). The extracellular domains of the glycoprotein hormones share moderate sequence similarity and contain a repeated series of conserved 25-residue leucine-rich motifs (reviewed in 32). These leucine-rich motifs may be important in protein-protein interactions in the binding of hormone to receptor. The membrane-spanning domains of the FSH, LH/CG, and TSH receptors have considerable sequence homology among themselves and with other members of the G-protein-coupled receptor family (32).

Knowledge of the structures of the genes for the receptors in this G-protein-coupled family can provide clues as to the functional differences and similarities as well as to the evolution of the genes. The gene structures of the α- and β-adrenergic receptors (23, 31), D1 and D2 dopamine receptors (24, 25), several muscarinic receptors (33), the putative G-21 protein (23), and rhodopsin (34) have been characterized. Genes for some of these receptors (adrenergic receptors, the D1 dopamine receptor, and the G-21 protein) contain no introns. However, rhodopsin and the dopamine D2 receptor genes have several introns within the coding region of the protein. The structures of the *LH receptor* (LH-R), *TSH receptor* (TSH-R), and FSH-R genes are more complex than the genes of other members in this receptor family (35–39).

We have characterized the FSH-R gene and its promoter (35). The FSH-R gene is very large, encompassing at least 85 kb of DNA that is divided into 10 exons often separated by very large introns (Fig. 8.1). The first 9 exons are relatively small and code for the amino terminal extracellular domain that contains the leucine repeat regions. The region of the molecule that encodes the 7 transmembrane-spanning regions is

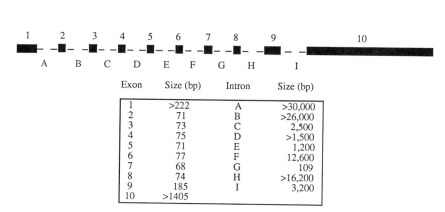

FIGURE 8.1. Basic organization of the FSH-R gene. The exons are drawn to scale and are numbered 1–10. The introns are abridged and lettered A–I. Exons 2–9 code for leucine-rich repeat sequences, and exon 10 codes for the entire transmembrane domain. The total size of the gene is estimated to be at least 85 kb. Adapted from Heckert, Daley, and Griswold (35).

contained within a single large exon (exon 10). The genes coding for FSH-R, TSH-R, and LH-R have a number of similarities: (i) They are all very large genes with 10 (TSH-R and FSH-R) or 11 (LH-R) exons; (ii) the last exon in each gene codes for the entire membrane-spanning region; and (iii) exons 2–9 code for the amino terminal repeats. This structure suggests that these genes arose from a single gene in which an exon coding for the leucine repeats was duplicated several times and was subsequently combined with the conserved exon for the transmembrane region. It has been proposed that these receptors (FSH-R, LH-R, and TSH-R) constitute a closely related subfamily of the G-protein-coupled receptors that have a relatively recent evolutionary origin (32).

## Expression of FSH-R in Sertoli and Granulosa Cells

The availability of cDNA probes for FSH-R has led to studies designed to localize the sites of synthesis and to examine the steady state levels of mRNA. Cloned genomic DNA corresponding to part of exon 10 of the FSH-R gene has been used as a probe on Northern blots to quantify the mRNA for FSH-R. We initially reported that Sertoli cells, ovary, and testis were found to contain a major transcript of 2.6 kb and a minor transcript of 4.5 kb that hybridized to the FSH-R DNA sequence (40, 41). Our preliminary analysis of these two transcripts indicates that the 4.5-kb transcript may have an extended 3' terminus, suggesting a possible alternative poly(A) addition site. If this proves to be the case, the protein product from each transcript would be identical. In a report from a different laboratory, the Northern blot analysis of ovarian mRNA revealed two major bands reported to be 7.0 and 2.5 kb (42). A third group has shown that the ovarian FSH-R mRNA consists of two transcripts of 2.6 and ~5 kb, which confirms our initial report (43). Camp et al. used in situ hybridization to show that FSH-R mRNA was localized exclusively in the granulosa cells in the ovary (43).

In the adult male rat, the expression of FSH-R is very dynamic, undergoing a cyclic change in steady state levels (40). Spermatogenesis in the adult rat is organized into a series of 14 stages that constitute the cycle of the seminiferous epithelium and that are defined by the germinal cell composition of the tubules (44). In the normal rat the 14 stages are present simultaneously at different regions along the length of the tubule, and the release of spermatozoa (spermiation) that occurs at stage VIII is asynchronous. There is good evidence that the functions of the Sertoli cells vary with the different stages of the cycle. We have utilized a scheme of retinol deprivation and repletion that results in the synchronization of the testis to 3 or 4 related stages of the cycle (45, 46). Spermatogenesis appears to proceed normally, but since the entire testis is in roughly the same stages, spermiation occurs only every 12–13 days. We have utilized the retinol synchronization method to obtain synchronized testes that represent all parts of the cycle. This method allows the collection of sufficient amounts of stage-synchronized testis to enable the analysis of low-abundance cell products (47).

We have speculated that the function of FSH in the adult rat may be confined to very discrete regions of the cycle of the seminiferous epithelium. Utilizing the FSH-R cDNA probe and mRNA isolated from synchronized testes, we were able to measure the steady state levels of FSH-R mRNA during the different stages of the cycle of the seminiferous epithelium (40). The mRNA was isolated from the testes of stage-synchronized rats and analyzed by Northern blots. We found that the relative levels of FSH-R mRNA varied in a cyclic manner, with low levels in stages V–IX and 5-fold-higher levels in stages XIII, XIV, and I. This result correlated very well to recent data from other laboratories that used the dissection method to determine other parameters of FSH action. The binding of labeled FSH and the ability of FSH to stimulate cAMP production were determined in dissected tubules of defined stages (48, 49). The tubules in stages XIII–II bound more FSH and responded to exogenous FSH with increased cAMP levels. The tubules in stages VII–VIII were essentially refractory to FSH stimulation of cAMP levels. Altogether, these studies suggest that the primary action of FSH in the adult male rat is cyclic in nature and may be confined to stages XII–IV.

## FSH or cAMP Regulation of FSH-R Gene Expression

Some initial reports have begun to appear that focus on the factors that regulate the expression of FSH-R in vivo. Sertoli cells treated in culture with FSH or cAMP showed a nearly complete down-regulation of FSH-R mRNA within 4 h (50). The action of FSH or cAMP did not result from the stimulation of FSH-R mRNA transcription, but appeared to be a result of a posttranscriptional mechanism. Experiments on ovarian function in vivo have shown that PMSG or FSH at low levels will stimulate follicular growth and increase the number of FSH-Rs and the steady state levels of FSH-R mRNA (42, 43). Higher concentrations of FSH (ovulatory levels) led to rapid decreases in the receptor mRNA within 12 h (42). Thus, at the level of the ovary, FSH and cAMP can lead to either increases or decreases in FSH-R mRNA depending on the different stages of follicular development.

## 5' Flanking Region of FSH-R Gene

Understanding the regulation of FSH-R mRNA at the transcriptional level involves an analysis of the promoter regions associated with the

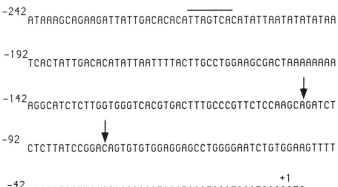

FIGURE 8.2. Sequence of 5' flanking region of FSH-R gene. The translational start site is designated as +1, and the transcriptional start sites are noted with an arrow. A consensus AP-1 site is marked with a line.

gene. We have characterized the 5' flanking region of the FSH-R gene (35) (Fig. 8.2). Primer extension and S1 nuclease experiments revealed the presence of two major transcriptional start sites at positions −80 and −98 relative to the translational start site. The promoter region immediately upstream from the transcriptional start site did not contain conventional TATA or CCAAT elements. The promoter did contain a consensus AP-1 binding site at position −214. AP-1 is a transcriptional factor that interacts with the promoters of phorbol ester-inducible genes. There is evidence that treatment of Sertoli cells with phorbol esters in culture results in a decreased response of the cells to FSH (51). The promoter region has characteristics that are similar to promoters of genes coding for "housekeeping" functions (52). Characteristics of these promoters include multiple transcription initiation sites, absence of TATA and CCAAT boxes, and high GC content. The 5' flanking regions of the LH-R gene and the TSH-R gene have also been sequenced and show similar characteristics. The sequences of these promoter regions have a higher overall GC content than does the corresponding region of the FSH-R gene (38, 39, 53).

This promoter is of considerable interest since it should contain cell-specific enhancer elements that allow expression of transgenes in Sertoli cells or granulosa cells. We constructed several fusion genes containing from 280 bp to 5 kbp of DNA 5' to the translational start site linked to the reporter gene *chloramphenicol acetyl transferase* (CAT) (Fig. 8.3). These gene constructs were transfected into cultured Sertoli cells, COS-7 cells, and a murine cell line derived from Sertoli cells designated as MSC-1. All these constructs actively promoted transcription of the reporter gene in primary cultures of Sertoli cells and MSC-1 cells, but not in COS-7 cells.

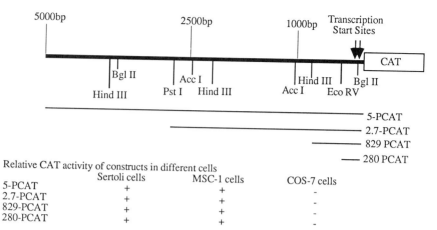

FIGURE 8.3. Partial restriction map and constructs on which preliminary data were obtained. The region 5' to the FSH-R gene was cloned into the plasmid pCAT-basic (Promega) that contains the reporter gene CAT. Immediately 5' to the CAT gene is ~60 bp of the 5' untranslated region of the FSH-R gene (30 bp upstream from ATG start codon). The constructs we have made are shown along with a partial restriction map and include promoter fragments of 5000, 2700, 829, and 280 bp. The activity of each of the constructs in Sertoli cells, MSC-1 cells, and primary cultures of Sertoli cells is summarized.

These results suggest that the DNA elements responsible for cell-specific transcription reside in the first 280 bp of the 5' flanking region. These initial results on the activity of the FSH-R gene promoter correlate well with data on the TSH-R promoter activity (53). It is likely, however, that future studies will reveal the regulation of the promoter regions of the FSH-R gene promoter to be extremely complex.

## References

1. Amsterdam A, Rotmensch S. Structure-function relationships during granulosa cell differentiation. Endocr Rev 1987;8(3):309–37.
2. Richards JS. Maturation of ovarian follicles: actions and interactions of pituitary and ovarian hormones on follicular cell differentiation. Physiol Rev 1980;60(1):51–89.
3. Hsueh AJW, Schaeffer JM. Gonadotropin-releasing hormone as a paracrine hormone and neurotransmitter in extra-pituitary sites. J Steroid Biochem 1985;23(5B):757–64.
4. Griswold MD, Morales C, Sylvester SR. Molecular biology of the Sertoli cell. Oxf Rev Reprod Biol 1988;10(124):124–61.
5. Griswold MD. Protein secretions of Sertoli cells. Int Rev Cytol 1988;110(133): 133–56.

6. Means AR, Dedman JR, Tindall DJ, Welsh MJ. Hormonal regulation of Sertoli cells. In: Endocrine approach to male contraception. Copenhagen: Scriptor, 1978:403–23.
7. Hseuh AJW, Adashi EY, Jones PBC, Welsh TH. Hormonal regulation of the differentiation of cultured granulosa cells. Endocr Rev 1984;5(1):76–127.
8. Means AR. Mechanisms of action of follicle-stimulating hormone (FSH). In: Johnson AD, Gomes WR, eds. The testis. New York: Academic Press, 1977:163–88.
9. Means AR, Dedman JR, Tash JS, Tindall DJ, van Sickle M, Welsh MJ. Regulation of the testis Sertoli cell by follicle-stimulating hormone. Annu Rev Physiol 1980;42(59):59–70.
10. Grasso P, Reichert LJ. Follicle-stimulating hormone receptor-mediated uptake of 45Ca2+ by proteoliposomes and cultured rat Sertoli cells: evidence for involvement of voltage-activated and voltage-independent calcium channels. Endocrinology 1989;125(6):3029–36.
11. Grasso P, Joseph MP, Reichert LE. A new role for follicle-stimulating hormone in the regulation of calcium flux in Sertoli cells: inhibition of $Na^+/Ca^{++}$ exchange. Endocrinology 1991;128(1):158–64.
12. Fritz IB. Comparison of granulosa and Sertoli cells at various stages of maturation: similarities and differences. Adv Exp Med Biol 1982;147(357):357–84.
13. Russell LD, Tallon DM, Weber JE, Wong V, Peterson RN. Three-dimensional reconstruction of a rat stage V Sertoli cell, III. A study of specific cellular relationships. Am J Anat 1983;167(2):181–92.
14. Russell LD. Normal testicular structure and methods for evaluation under experimental and disruptive conditions. In: Clarkson TW, Nordberg GF, Sager PR, eds. Reproductive and developmental toxicity of metals. New York: Plenum Press, 1983:227–52.
15. Russell LD, Peterson RN. Determination of the elongate spermatid-Sertoli cell ratio in various mammals. J Reprod Fertil 1984;70(2):635–41.
16. Russell LD, Bartke A, Goh JC. Postnatal development of the Sertoli cell barrier, tubular lumen, and cytoskeleton of Sertoli and myoid cells in the rat, and their relationship to tubular fluid secretion and flow. Am J Anat 1989;184(3):179–89.
17. Orth JM. Proliferation of Sertoli cells in fetal and postnatal rats: a quantitative autoradiographic study. Anat Rec 1982;203(4):485–92.
18. Orth JM. The role of follicle-stimulating hormone in controlling Sertoli cell proliferation in testes of fetal rats. Endocrinology 1984;115(4):1248–55.
19. Parmentier M. Molecular cloning of the thyrotropin receptor. Science 1989;246:1620–2.
20. Loosfelt H, Misrahi M, Atger M, et al. Cloning and sequencing of porcine LH-hCG receptor cDNA: variants lacking transmembrane domain. Science 1989;245:525–8.
21. McFarland KC, Sprengel R, Phillips HS, et al. Lutropin-choriogonadotropin receptor: an unusual member of the G protein-coupled receptor family. Science 1989;245:494–9.
22. Sprengel R, Braun T, Nikolics K, Segaloff DL, Seeburg PH. The testicular receptor for follicle stimulating hormone: structure and functional expression of cloned cDNA. Mol Endocrinol 1990;4(4):525–30.

23. Kobilka BK, Frielle T, Collins S, et al. An intronless gene encoding a potential member of the family of receptors coupled to guanine nucleotide regulatory protein. Nature 1987;329:75–9.
24. Dal Toso R, Sommer B, Ewert M, et al. The dopamine D2 receptor: two molecular forms generated by alternative splicing. EMBO J 1989;8:4025–34.
25. Sunahara RK. Human dopamine D1 receptor encoded by an intronless gene on chromosome 5. Nature 1990;347:80–3.
26. O'Dowd BF, Lefkowitz RJ, Caron MG. Structure of the adrenergic and related receptors. Annu Rev Neurosci 1989;12:67–83.
27. Johnson GL, Dhanasedaran N. The G protein family and their interaction with receptors. Endocr Rev 1989;10:317–31.
28. Gocayne J, Robinson DA, Fitzgerald MG, et al. Primary structure of rat cardiac β-adrenergic and muscarinic cholinergic receptors obtained by automated DNA sequence analysis: further evidence for a multi-gene family. Proc Natl Acad Sci USA 1987;84:8296–300.
29. Bunzow JR, Van Tol HHM, Grandy DK, et al. Cloning and expression of the rat D2 dopamine receptor. Nature 1988;336:783–7.
30. Kobilka BK, Frielle T, Dohlman HG, et al. The delineation of the intronless nature of the genes for the human and hamster β2-adrenergic receptor and their putative promoter regions. J Biol Chem 1987;262:7321–7.
31. Kobilka BK, Matsui H, Kobilka T, et al. Cloning and expression of the gene coding for the human platelet alpha-2 adrenergic receptor. Science 1987; 238:650–6.
32. Vassart G, Parmentier M, Libert F, Dumont J. Molecular genetics of the thyrotropin receptor. Trends Endocrinol Metab 1991;2(4):151–6.
33. Bonner TI, Buckley NJ, Young AC, Brann MR. Identification of a family of muscarinic acetylcholine receptor genes. Science 1987;237:527–32.
34. Nathans J, Hogness DS. Isolation, sequence analysis and intron-exon arrangement of the gene encoding bovine rhodopsin. Cell 1983;34:807–14.
35. Heckert LL, Daley I, Griswold MD. Structural organization of the follicle hormone receptor gene. Mol Endocrinol 1992;6:70–80.
36. Gross B, Misrahi M, Sar S, Milgrom E. Composite structure of the human thyrotropin receptor gene. Biochem Biophys Res Commun 1991;177:679–87.
37. Tsai-Morris CH, Buczko E, Wang W, Dufau ML. Intronic nature of the rat luteinizing hormone receptor subspecies with hormone binding activity. J Biol Chem 1990;265(32):19385–8.
38. Tsai-Morris CH, Buczko E, Wei W, Xie XZ, Dufau ML. Structural organization of the rat luteinizing hormone (LH) receptor gene. J Biol Chem 1991;266:11355–8.
39. Koo YB, Ji I, Slaughter RG, Ji TH. Structure of the luteinizing hormone receptor gene and multiple exons of the coding sequence. Endocrinology 1991;128:2297–650.
40. Heckert LL, Griswold MD. Expression of follicle-stimulating hormone receptor mRNA in rat testes and Sertoli cells. Mol Endocrinol 1991;5(5): 670–7.
41. Heckert LL, Griswold MD. Expression of the FSH receptor in the testis. Recent Prog Horm Res 1992.
42. LaPolt PS, Tilly JL, Aihara T, Nishimori K, Hsueh A. Gonadotropin-induced up- and down-regulation of ovarian follicle stimulating hormone (FSH)

receptor gene expression in immature rats: effects of pregnant mare's serum gonadotropin, human chorionic gonadotropin and recombinant FSH. Endocrinology 1992;130(3):1289–95.
43. Camp TA, Rahal JO, Mayo KE. Cellular localization and hormonal regulation of follicle-stimulating hormone and luteinizing hormone receptor messenger RNAs in the rat ovary. Mol Endocrinol 1991;5:1405–17.
44. Leblond CP, Clermont Y. Definition of the stages of the cycle of the seminiferous epithelium in the rat. Ann N Y Acad Sci 1952;55:548–73.
45. Morales CR, Griswold MD. Retinol induces stage synchronization in seminiferous tubules of vitamin A deficient rats. Ann of N Y Acad Sci 1987;513:292–3.
46. Morales C, Hugly S, Griswold MD. Stage-dependent levels of specific mRNA transcripts in Sertoli cells. Biol Reprod 1987;36(4):1035–46.
47. Morales CR, Alcivar AA, Hecht NB, Griswold MD. Specific mRNAs in Sertoli and germinal cells of testes from stage synchronized rats. Mol Endocrinol 1989;3(4):725–33.
48. Kangasniemi M, Kaipia A, Toppari J, Perheentupa A, Huhtaniemi I, Parvinen M. Cellular regulation of follicle-stimulating hormone (FSH) binding in rat seminiferous tubules. J Androl 1990;11(4):336–43.
49. Kangasniemi M, Kaipia A, Mali P, Toppari J, Huhtaniemi I, Parvinen M. Modulation of basal and FSH-dependent cyclic AMP production in rat seminiferous tubules staged by an improved transillumination technique. Anat Rec 1990;227(1):62–76.
50. Themmen A, Blok L, Post M, et al. Follitropin receptor down regulation involves a cAMP-dependent post-transcriptional decrease of receptor mRNA expression. Mol Cell Endocrinol 1991;78:R7–13.
51. Monaco L, Conti M. Inhibition by phorbol esters and other tumor promoters of the response of the Sertoli cell to FSH: evidence for dual site of action. Mol Cell Endocrinol 1987;49(2–3):227–36.
52. Dynan WS. Promoters for housekeeping genes. Trends Genet 1986;2:196–7.
53. Ikuyama S, Niller H, Shimura H, Akamizu T, Kohn LD. Characterization of the 5'-flanking region of the rat thyrotropin receptor gene. Mol Endocrinol 1992;6:793–804.

# 9
# Mouse Ovarian Prolactin Receptors

DIANA L. CLARKE, KATHLEEN H. YOUNG, AND DANIEL I.H. LINZER

Pituitary *prolactin* (PRL) is a protein hormone with a broad range of physiological targets, including the ovary. The pituitary is not the only origin of PRL-like activity, though. Other hormones, including human decidual-derived PRL (1, 2) and rat decidual luteotropin (3), are also able to bind to the PRL receptor with similar affinities. In the mouse, rat, hamster, cow, sheep, and human, placental-derived hormones are produced that bind to the PRL receptor (4). These *placental lactogens* (PL) are the predominant hormones with PRL-like activity in the circulation during mid- to late pregnancy. Two PLs are synthesized in rodents, and they are designated as *placental lactogen I* (PL-I) and *placental lactogen II* (PL-II). High levels of PL-I accumulate transiently at midgestation (5), and the appearance of PL-I in the maternal serum coincides with a cessation of the early gestational surges of PRL release from the pituitary (6). PL-II synthesis is first detected at midpregnancy, and unlike PL-I, PL-II levels increase until parturition (7).

The actions of PRL and the other hormones with PRL-like activity are initiated by binding of the hormone to cell-surface PRL receptors. The PRL receptor, although a single polypeptide chain, is actually several distinct proteins that arise by alternative mRNA splicing (8–10). These proteins span the plasma membrane once, indicating that they have distinct modes of action from the 7-transmembrane domain, G-protein-linked gonadotropin receptors. The initial isolate of a PRL receptor cDNA clone predicted a protein with a relatively short cytoplasmic domain (8); subsequent cDNA clones identified differences in sequence among the various PRL receptors that occur exclusively in the carboxy-terminal region of the cytoplasmic domain, resulting in additional short (9) or long (10) receptor forms. Thus, binding of a common ligand to the different receptor forms can activate distinct intracellular signaling pathways. To date, PRL signaling has only been demonstrated to occur through the receptor form with a long cytoplasmic domain, leading to transcriptional activation of a milk protein gene promoter in transfected cell cultures (11). However, the PRL receptors, including the long-form receptor, lack any obvious signal transduction motifs (e.g., nucleotide binding or protein kinase domains), and a signaling pathway common to all PRL target cell types has not been identified.

One of the principal targets of PRL (and of PL-I and PL-II) is the ovary, and the effects of PRL on the corpus luteum were reflected in the early naming of PRL as *hypophysial luteotrophin* (12). PRL is a critical regulator of follicular development during the reproductive cycle and of the formation, maintenance, and functioning of the corpus luteum. This hormone is instrumental for a blockade of prostaglandin PGF-2α-induced (13–15) or LH-induced (16, 17) luteolysis in rodents, but under some circumstances PRL can also promote luteolysis (18, 19). Numerous molecular effects of PRL on the ovary have been described, including the maintenance of increased *luteinizing hormone* (LH) receptor levels in luteal and granulosa cells (20, 21); increased synthesis of $\alpha_2$-macroglobulin, which is involved in remodeling of the ovary during granulosa cell differentiation (22); and increased or decreased steroidogenesis. PRL stimulates an increase in ovarian progesterone production by regulating the levels of both biosynthetic enzymes for progesterone precursors as well as enzymes that modify progesterone to inactive forms (19, 23–25).

In contrast to the stimulation of progesterone synthesis and stability, PRL generally inhibits estradiol synthesis by blocking the follicle stimulating hormone-induced increase in aromatase mRNA and protein levels (25–31). However, at midpregnancy PL-I has been implicated in increasing aromatase levels (30, 31). Thus, the response of the ovary to PRL (or PL) can vary. This variable responsiveness may depend on the presence of other cooperating or interfering hormones, but may also involve differences between PRL and PL-I or changes in the forms, locations, or amounts of the PRL receptors in the ovary. We therefore sought to determine if all four of the mouse PRL receptor mRNAs are expressed in the ovary and how expression of these forms changes during pregnancy. In addition, to identify potential components of the PRL receptor signaling pathway(s), we have begun to search for intracellular proteins that interact with the cytoplasmic domains of the distinct PRL receptor forms.

## Results and Discussion

### PRL Receptor Forms in the Mouse Ovary

Four forms of the PRL receptor have been isolated as cDNA clones of mouse liver mRNAs (Fig. 9.1). Three of these mRNAs encode receptor proteins with relatively short cytoplasmic domains, which are therefore

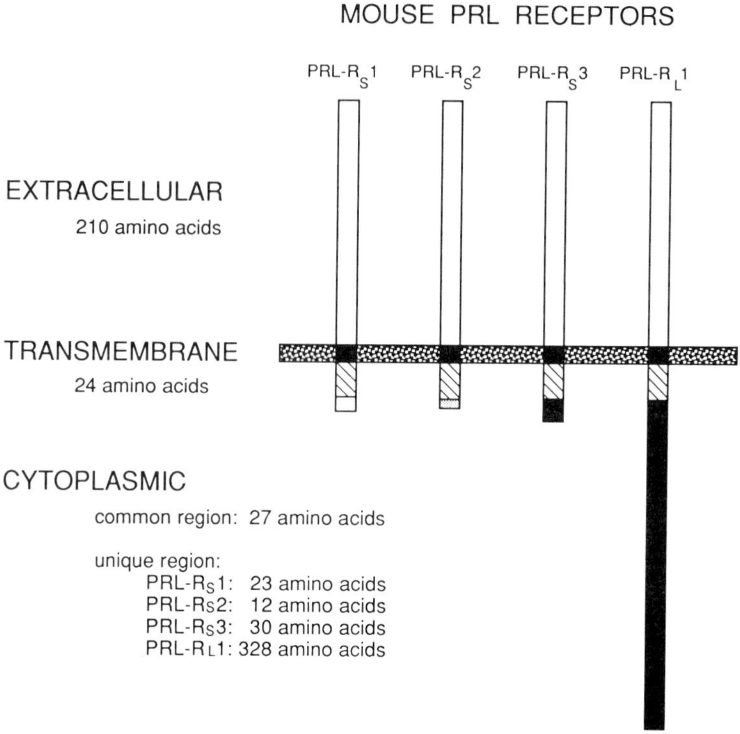

## MOUSE PRL RECEPTORS

PRL-R$_S$1  PRL-R$_S$2  PRL-R$_S$3  PRL-R$_L$1

EXTRACELLULAR
210 amino acids

TRANSMEMBRANE
24 amino acids

CYTOPLASMIC
common region: 27 amino acids

unique region:
PRL-R$_S$1: 23 amino acids
PRL-R$_S$2: 12 amino acids
PRL-R$_S$3: 30 amino acids
PRL-R$_L$1: 328 amino acids

FIGURE 9.1. Schematic diagram of mouse PRL receptors. Each of the 4 receptor forms is a single polypeptide chain with identical extracellular (open box), transmembrane (solid box), and membrane-proximal cytoplasmic (hatched box) domains. The sequences of the 4 receptors diverge at the same point in the cytoplasmic domain, giving rise to distinct carboxytermini. The structures of the 3 short forms are reported in reference 35; the structure of the mouse PRL receptor long form is from Clarke and Linzer (unpublished observations).

designated PRL-R$_S$1, PRL-R$_S$2, and PRL-R$_S$3, while one mRNA encodes a protein, PRL-R$_l$1, with a long cytoplasmic domain; only one short form has been reported for other species, which closely resembles mouse PRL-R$_S$3 (8, 9). Attempts to identify PRL receptor mRNAs in tissues other than the liver by filter hybridization have proven difficult due to the low abundance of these mRNAs (9). We have therefore utilized a combined *reverse transcription/polymerase chain reaction* (RT/PCR) approach to determine if all four receptor forms are expressed in the mouse ovary.

Ovary and liver RNAs were subjected to RT/PCR using random primers to synthesize the single-stranded cDNA and oligonucleotide primers from the unique sequences of each receptor mRNA for PCR amplification; $^{32}$P-dATP was included during the reaction to enable

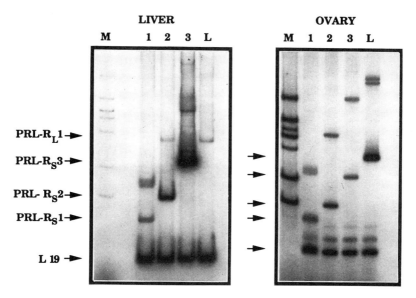

FIGURE 9.2. RT/PCR analysis of PRL receptor mRNAs in the mouse liver and ovary. Total liver and ovary RNAs were reverse transcribed using random primer oligonucleotides and 1 μg of RNA. Each of the 2 cDNA reactions were then divided equally into 4 samples, supplemented with $^{32}$P-dATP and oligonucleotide primer pairs specific for each receptor mRNA or for the L19 ribosomal protein mRNA, and amplified by 20 PCR cycles. Products were electrophoresed on a 6% polyacrylamide gel and autoradiographed. The arrows indicate the products of the expected size; higher molecular weight products may represent amplification of precursor RNAs. (M = markers; 1 = PRL-$R_S$1; 2 = PRL-$R_S$2; 3 = PRL-$R_S$3; L = PRL-$R_L$1.)

detection of the products by polyacrylamide gel electrophoresis and autoradiography (Fig. 9.2). Included in each reaction was a pair of oligonucleotide primers for the L19 ribosomal protein mRNA, which serves as an internal control (32; the oligonucleotides were designed from the sequence of the mouse L19 mRNA, GenBank accession number M62952). Examination of the reaction products reveals that all four forms of PRL receptor mRNA are synthesized in both the mouse liver and ovary. However, whereas the PRL-$R_S$3 mRNA is the most abundant form in the liver, the PRL-$R_L$1 mRNA is more abundant than the other three forms in the ovary. Thus, PRL receptor expression may be regulated by tissue-specific differences in RNA processing or in mRNA degradation rates, leading to variations in the relative amounts of the four receptor forms.

RNA was prepared from ovaries at various days of gestation and during lactation and again analyzed by RT/PCR. Reactions were carried out with varying amounts of RNA and for varying numbers of PCR cycles

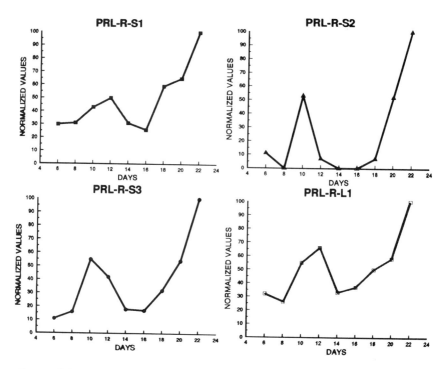

FIGURE 9.3. Mouse ovarian PRL receptor mRNA levels during gestation. Ovary RNAs were prepared from various days of gestation and lactation. These RNAs were analyzed by RT/PCR as described in Figure 9.2. Autoradiograms of the RT/PCR products were quantified using a phosphorimager, and receptor levels were normalized to the L19 ribosomal protein mRNA internal control. The maximal amount of each receptor mRNA is arbitrarily assigned a value of 100. For comparison, the level of PRL-$R_L$1 mRNA at day 10 is approximately 2-fold, 4-fold, and 20-fold greater than the mRNA levels of PRL-$R_S$3, PRL-$R_S$1, and PRL-$R_S$2, respectively.

to ensure that the analysis was conducted in the linear range for each PRL receptor mRNA. Resultant autoradiograms were quantified, and receptor mRNA levels were normalized against the L19 internal control (Fig. 9.3). All four mRNAs were found to increase in amount transiently at midgestation, then to decline to levels present in early pregnancy, and finally to increase again steadily from day 16 of gestation through term and during lactation. At day 10, PRL-$R_L$1 levels are approximately 2-fold, 4-fold, and 20-fold greater than those of PRL-$R_S$3, PRL-$R_S$1, and PRL-$R_S$2, respectively. The pattern of changes in receptor mRNA levels during gestation is similar to that seen for the circulating levels of receptor ligand, with the relatively low levels of PRL during early pregnancy replaced by a dramatic and transient increase in serum mPL-I at midpregnancy, followed by a steady increase in mPL-II levels from midpregnancy until term (4). Thus, the changes in PRL receptor mRNA levels in the ovary may reflect ligand-induced up- and down-regulation of receptor expression.

The analysis of receptor mRNA levels does not necessarily indicate that each of the four receptor forms is present in the same cell type in the ovary. To identify the sites of synthesis of the various PRL receptors in the ovary, we therefore prepared $^{35}$S-labeled single-stranded RNA probes by in vitro transcription of the cDNA clones and used these probes for in situ hybridization to ovary sections. Furthermore, while the extremely low levels of PRL receptor mRNA might preclude straightforward detection by filter hybridization, the localization of receptor mRNA in a subset of ovarian cell types and structures might significantly enhance the sensitivity of the in situ hybridization approach.

Our initial attempts to detect the PRL receptor mRNA in the ovary by in situ hybridization utilized a probe from the region of the mRNA common to all four forms, which should provide the strongest hybrid-

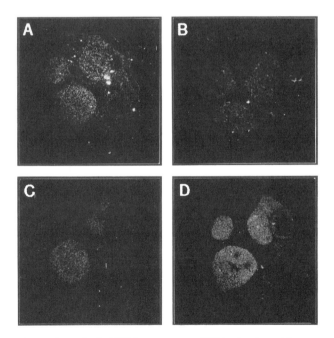

FIGURE 9.4. Detection of all 4 PRL receptor mRNAs in the midpregnant mouse ovary. Gestational day-10 ovaries were sectioned and hybridized to $^{35}$S-labeled antisense probes generated from the unique (coding and 3' noncoding) regions of each of the 4 PRL receptor cDNAs. Shown are dark-field photomicrographs with light regions indicating hybridization. (A = PRL-R$_S$1; B = PRL-R$_S$2; C = PRL-R$_S$3; D = PRL-R$_L$1.)

ization signal. Using this probe, total receptor mRNA is detectable and is found localized to the corpus luteum, granulosa cells of large follicles, and interstitial cells in the nonpregnant ovary (data not shown). Hybridization experiments were then repeated using ovary sections from mice at various days of gestation and probes generated by transcription of the unique regions of each of the four receptor mRNAs. These studies reveal that at midpregnancy (gestational day 10), all four PRL receptor mRNAs can be detected primarily, if not exclusively, within the corpus luteum (Fig. 9.4); hybridization is not detected at significant levels within follicles at this time.

Comparison of in situ hybridizations to ovary sections from various times in gestation reveals that all four receptor mRNAs are expressed in the corpus luteum throughout pregnancy, but that expression in follicles increases in late pregnancy. In addition, increases and decreases in receptor mRNA levels can be detected by in situ hybridization that closely follow the quantitative RT/PCR results. An example of these data is shown for the PRL-$R_L$1 mRNA (Fig. 9.5), which also reveals that receptor synthesis in follicles is restricted to the granulosa cells. Furthermore, PRL receptor mRNA is not detected in all follicles, con-

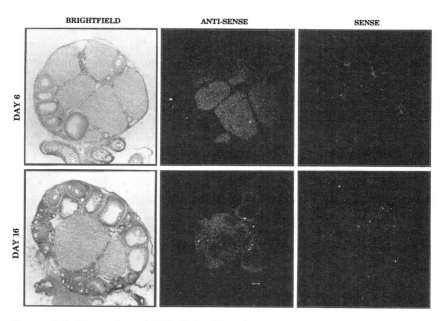

FIGURE 9.5. Expression of PRL-$R_L$1 mRNA in the mouse ovary in early and late pregnancy. Ovaries from day 6 (top) and day 16 (bottom) of gestation were sectioned and hybridized to $^{35}$S-labeled sense or antisense probes from the unique region of the PRL-$R_L$1 mRNA. Shown from left to right are bright-field photomicrographs of the ovary section, dark-field views of the antisense probe hybridization, and dark-field images of the sense hybridization.

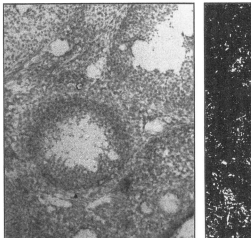
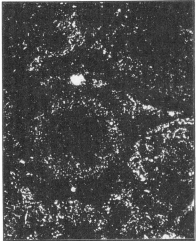

FIGURE 9.6. Expression of PRL-$R_S2$ mRNA in small follicles. Gestational day-8 ovaries were sectioned and hybridized with the PRL-$R_S2$ antisense probe. Shown are the bright-field (left) and dark-field (right) views. Hybridization can be seen as light regions within the granulosa cell layer of the small follicle in the center of the photomicrograph.

sistent with receptor expression occurring only in those healthy follicles that may continue to develop and ovulate in the next reproductive cycle. Subtle differences in the patterns of expression of the four receptor mRNAs in follicles during gestation can be seen, however, and presumably reflect a regulation of PRL receptor expression at a posttranscriptional level. For example, the PRL-$R_S2$ mRNA is the only receptor mRNA detected in small, and perhaps atretic, follicles at day 8 of gestation, suggesting a specific role for this receptor form in this class of follicles (Fig. 9.6).

## Interactions of PRL Receptor Cytoplasmic Domains with Cellular Proteins

To search for cellular proteins that may be involved in PRL receptor signal transduction, receptor cytoplasmic domains (without the extracellular or transmembrane domains) were generated as bacterial fusion proteins and used as affinity reagents. The cytoplasmic domain coding regions of the four receptor mRNAs were inserted into the pGEX3X vector (33) in frame with the upstream sequences encoding *glutathione-S-transferase* (GST). The GST-PRL receptor cytoplasmic domain fusion proteins were purified from bacterial cell lysates by binding to glutathione agarose beads. Since the GST portion of the fusion protein would be

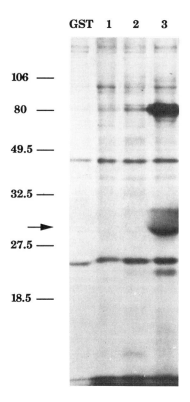

FIGURE 9.7. Binding of HC11 mammary epithelial cell proteins to the short PRL receptor cytoplasmic domains. $^{35}$S-labeled proteins extracted from HC11 cells were incubated with agarose beads containing GST alone or the GST-PRL receptor cytoplasmic domain fusion proteins for PRL-R$_S$1 (lane 1), PRL-R$_S$2 (lane 2), or PRL-R$_S$3 (lane 3). Bound proteins were eluted with glutathione and visualized by gel electrophoresis and autoradiography. The arrow indicates the 30-kd polypeptide that binds specifically to the PRL-R$_S$3 cytoplasmic domain.

bound to the beads, we reasoned that this would select for proteins that had folded properly (at least for the GST domain) and would position the receptor cytoplasmic domain so that it was free to interact with other proteins. These beads were then incubated with $^{35}$S-methionine/cysteine-labeled lysates of PRL-responsive cell lines. After washing the beads, bound proteins were eluted by addition of glutathione and analyzed by polyacrylamide gel electrophoresis.

HC11 mouse mammary epithelial cells, which respond to PRL by synthesizing milk proteins (34), represented one source of radiolabeled cell lysates. Analysis of HC11 proteins bound to the GST-PRL receptor beads reveals the binding of a 30-kd polypeptide specifically to the PRL-R$_S$3 fusion protein (Fig. 9.7); binding of this polypeptide to GST alone or to GST fusion proteins with the other short-receptor-form cytoplasmic domains is not detected (Fig. 9.7), and binding is also not detected to GST fusions with the PRL-$R_L1$ cytoplasmic domain or with unrelated proteins (data not shown). Additional polypeptides of 78 kd and 22 kd that appear to bind preferentially to the GST-PRL-$R_S3$ fusion protein are found in other experiments to bind to other fusion proteins as well

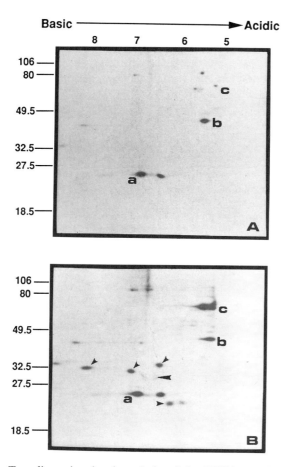

FIGURE 9.8. Two-dimensional gel analysis of the HC11 proteins bound to the PRL-$R_S3$ cytoplasmic domain. $^{35}$S-labeled HC11 proteins bound and eluted from agarose beads containing GST alone (A) or the GST-PRL-$R_S3$ cytoplasmic domain (B) were analyzed by two-dimensional gel electrophoresis. The small, diagonal arrows point to the 3 specifically bound polypeptides; the large arrow indicates the position of the unlabeled fusion protein eluted from the beads along with the radiolabeled HC11 proteins; the small horizontal arrow highlights the 22-kd polypeptide that appears to bind PRL-$R_S3$ specifically, but is in fact seen with other fusion proteins as well; and spots a, b, and c are used for alignment of the two autoradiograms.

(including fusion proteins unrelated to the PRL receptor) and are therefore considered unlikely to be involved in PRL receptor function.

The 30-kd protein bound to the PRL-$R_S$3 cytoplasmic domain forms a diffuse band due to the presence of large amounts of the eluted GST-PRL receptor fusion protein—which is predicted to be 31 kd—in the sample. We therefore analyzed the HC11 proteins bound and eluted from the GST-PRL-$R_S$3 fusion protein by two-dimensional gel electrophoresis as well. By this technique the 30-kd polypeptide is separated from the unlabeled fusion protein and can be seen to resolve into three species of pI 6.7, 7.3, and 8.0 (Fig. 9.8). One possible explanation for the binding of the 78-kd doublet is that the fusion protein preparations vary in the amount of malfolded protein recognized by members of the heat shock

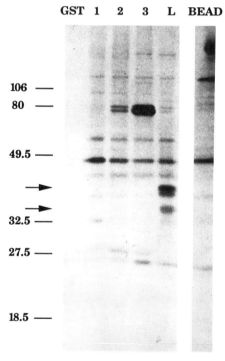

FIGURE 9.9. Binding of Nb2 lymphoma cell proteins to the 4 PRL receptor cytoplasmic domains. $^{35}$S-labeled proteins extracted from Nb2 cells were incubated with agarose beads containing GST alone or the GST-PRL receptor cytoplasmic domain fusion proteins for PRL-$R_S$1 (lane 1), PRL-$R_S$2 (lane 2), PRL-$R_S$3 (lane 3), or PRL-$R_L$1 (lane L). Bound proteins were eluted with glutathione and visualized by gel electrophoresis and autoradiography. Also shown are the residual proteins bound to the agarose beads containing GST alone after elution by glutathione (BEAD); residual proteins were removed by boiling in SDS sample buffer for gel analysis. The arrows indicate the 33- and 37-kd polypeptides that bind specifically to the PRL-$R_L$1 cytoplasmic domain.

family, which includes GRP78/BiP, a 78-kd protein in the endoplasmic reticulum that binds incorrectly folded proteins (36).

Binding experiments were also carried out with radiolabeled lysates of the Nb2 cell line (Fig. 9.9), a rat T cell lymphoma that is dependent upon PRL for proliferation (35). As previously observed with HC11 cell lysates, a doublet of 78 kd associates preferentially with the PRL-$R_S$3 fusion protein, but is again considered nonspecific because this doublet binds to other fusion proteins as well. No other Nb2 binding proteins specific for any of the short receptor forms are detected. However, two polypeptides of 33 and 37 kd are observed to bind specifically to the PRL-$R_L$1 cytoplasmic domain. The limited number of proteins found to bind specifically to the different forms of the PRL receptor suggests that these proteins may be relevant to PRL receptor signaling, regulation, or trafficking in the cell.

## Summary

All four forms of the mouse PRL receptor are expressed in both the liver and the ovary, but these two tissues display different relative levels of the four receptor mRNAs. In the ovary, receptor mRNA increases in amount at midgestation, then declines to a level equivalent to that in early pregnancy, and then increases to a high level at term and during lactation. The receptor mRNAs are detected in the corpus luteum, interstitial cells, and the granulosa cells of certain follicles. Expression in the corpus luteum continues throughout pregnancy, while granulosa cell expression appears to be restricted primarily to late gestation. This is most pronounced for PRL-$R_L$1 mRNA, which is the most abundant PRL receptor mRNA in the ovary. Using two PRL-responsive cell lines, three polypeptides with similar molecular weight and varying isoelectric points are found to bind specifically to the cytoplasmic domain of PRL-$R_S$3, while two polypeptides of approximately 33 and 37 kd are detected that bind only to the PRL-$R_L$1 cytoplasmic domain. These polypeptides may therefore participate in the functioning of individual forms of the PRL receptor.

*Acknowledgments.* This work was supported by a grant from the National Institutes of Health to D.I.H.L. (HD-24518). D.L.C. is a predoctoral trainee in the Reproductive Sciences Training Program; K.H.Y. received support from a National Institutes of Health postdoctoral fellowship; and D.I.H.L. is the recipient of an American Cancer Society Faculty Research Award.

## References

1. Riddick DH, Luciano AA, Kusmick WF, Maslar IA. De novo synthesis of prolactin by human decidua. Life Sci 1978;23:1913–21.
2. Golander A, Hurley T, Barrett J, Hizi A, Handwerger S. Prolactin synthesis by human chorion-decidual tissue: a possible source of prolactin in the amniotic fluid. Science 1978;202:311–3.
3. Jayatilak PG, Glaser LA, Basuray R, Kelly PA, Gibori G. Identification and partial characterization of a prolactin-like hormone produced by rat decidual tissue. Proc Natl Acad Sci USA 1985;82:217–21.
4. Ogren L, Talamantes F. Prolactins of pregnancy and their cellular source. Int Rev Cytol 1988;112:1–65.
5. Ogren L, Southard JN, Colosi P, Linzer DIH, Talamantes F. Mouse placental lactogen, I. RIA and gestational profile in maternal serum. Endocrinology 1989;125:2253–7.
6. Barkley MS, Radford GE, Geschwind II. The pattern of plasma prolactin concentration during the first half of mouse gestation. Biol Reprod 1978;19:291–6.
7. Soares MJ, Colosi PC, Talamantes F. Development and characterization of a homologous radioimmunoassay for mouse placental lactogen. Endocrinology 1982;110:668–70.
8. Boutin JM, Jolicoeur C, Okamura H, et al. Cloning and expression of the rat prolactin receptor, a member of the growth hormone/prolactin receptor gene family. Cell 1988;53:69–77.
9. Davis JA, Linzer DIH. Expression of multiple prolactin receptors in mouse liver. Mol Endocrinol 1989;3:674–80.
10. Edery M, Jolicoeur C, Levi-Meyrueis C, et al. Identification and sequence analysis of a second form of prolactin receptor by molecular cloning of complementary DNA from rabbit mammary gland. Proc Natl Acad Sci USA 1989;86:2112–6.
11. Lesueur L, Edery M, Ali S, Paly J, Kelly PA, Djiane J. Comparison of long and short forms of the prolactin receptor on prolactin-induced milk protein gene transcription. Proc Natl Acad Sci USA 1991;88:824–8.
12. Astwood EB. The regulation of corpus luteum function by hypophyseal luteotrophin. Endocrinology 1941;28:309–20.
13. Grinwich DL, Hichens M, Behrman HR. Control of the LH receptor by prolactin and prostaglandin F2α in rat corpora lutea. Biol Reprod 1976;14:212–8.
14. Behrman HR, Grinwich DL, Hichens M, MacDonald GJ. Effects of hypophysectomy, prolactin, and prostaglandin F2α on gonadotropin binding in vivo and in vitro in the corpus luteum. Endocrinology 1978;103:349–57.
15. Harris KH, Murphy BD. Luteolysis in the hamster: abrogation by gonadotropin and prolactin pretreatment. Prostaglandins 1981;21:177–87.
16. Sanchez-Criado JE, Lopez F, Aguilar E. Pituitary regulation of corpus luteum progesterone secretion in cyclic rats. Endocrinology 1986;119:1083–8.
17. Sanchez-Criado JE, Van der Schoot P, Uilenbroek JT. Evidence for luteotrophic and antiluteolytic actions of prolactin in rats with 5-day oestrous cycles. J Endocrinol 1988;117:455–60.

18. Richards JS, Williams JJ. Luteal cell receptor content for prolactin (PRL) and luteinizing hormone (LH): regulation by LH and PRL. Endocrinology 1976;99:1571–81.
19. Martel C, Labrie C, Dupont E, et al. Regulation of 3 beta-hydroxysteroid dehydrogenase/delta 5-delta 4 isomerase expression and activity in the hypophysectomized rat ovary: interactions between the stimulatory effect of human chorionic gonadotropin and the luteolytic effect of prolactin. Endocrinology 1990;127:2726–37.
20. Gibori G, Richards JS. Dissociation of two distinct luteotropic effects of prolactin: regulation of luteinizing hormone-receptor content and progesterone secretion during pregnancy. Endocrinology 1978;102:767–74.
21. Piquette GN, LaPolt PS, Oikawa M, Hsueh AJW. Regulation of luteinizing hormone receptor messenger ribonucleic acid levels by gonadotropins, growth factors, and gonadotropin-releasing hormone in cultured rat granulosa cells. Endocrinology 1991;128:2449–56.
22. Gaddy-Kurten D, Richards JS. Regulation of α2-macroglobulin by luteinizing hormone and prolactin during cell differentiation in the rat ovary. Mol Endocrinol 1991;5:1280–91.
23. Behrman HR, Orczyk GP, MacDonald GJ. Prolactin induction of enzymes controlling luteal cholesterol turnover. Endocrinology 1970;87:1251–6.
24. Jones PBC, Valk CA, Hsueh AJW. Regulation of progestin biosynthetic enzymes in cultured rat granulosa cells: effects of prolactin, $\beta_2$-adrenergic agonist, human chorionic gonadotropin and gonadotropin releasing hormone. Biol Reprod 1983;29:572–85.
25. Lamprecht SA, Lindner HR, Strauss JF. Induction of 20α-hydroxysteroid dehydrogenase in rat corpora lutea by pharmacological blockade of pituitary prolactin secretion. Biochim Biophys Acta 1969;187:133–43.
26. Wang C, Hsueh AJW, Erickson GF. Prolactin inhibition of estrogen production by cultured rat granulosa cells. Mol Cell Endocrinol 1980;20:135–44.
27. Tsai-Morris CH, Ghosh M, Hirshfield AN, Wise PM, Brodie AMH. Inhibition of ovarian aromatase by prolactin in vivo. Biol Reprod 1983;29:342–6.
28. Wang C, Chan V. Divergent effects of prolactin on estrogen and progesterone production by granulosa cells of rat graafian follicles. Endocrinology 1982;110:1085–93.
29. Dorrington J, Gore-Langton RE. Prolactin inhibits oestrogen synthesis in the ovary. Nature 1981;290:600–2.
30. Krasnow JS, Hickey GJ, Richards JS. Regulation of aromatase mRNA and estradiol biosynthesis in rat ovarian granulosa and luteal cells by prolactin. Mol Endocrinol 1990;4:12–13.
31. Hickey GJ, Oonk RB, Hall PF, Richards JS. Aromatase cytochrome P450 and cholesterol side-chain cleavage cytochrome P450 in corpora lutea of pregnant rats: diverse regulation by peptide and steroid hormones. Endocrinology 1989;125:1673–82.
32. Camp TA, Rahal JO, Mayo KE. Cellular localization and hormonal regulation of follicle-stimulating hormone and luteinizing hormone receptor messenger RNAs in the rat ovary. Mol Endocrinol 1991;5:1405–17.
33. Smith DB, Johnson KS. Single step purification of polypeptides expressed in *Escherichia coli* as fusions with glutathione-S-transferase. Gene 1988;67:31–40.

34. Ball RK, Frillis RR, Schoenenberger CA, Doppler W, Groner B. Prolactin regulation of β-casein gene expression and of a cytosolic 120-Kd protein in a cloned mouse mammary epithelial cell line. EMBO J 1988;7:2089–95.
35. Gout PW, Beer CT, Noble RL. Prolactin-stimulated growth of cell cultures established from malignant Nb rat lymphomas. Cancer Res 1980;40:2433–6.
36. Gething MJ, Sambrook J. Protein folding in the cell. Nature 1992;355:33–45.

# 10

# Molecular Regulation of Genes Involved in Ovulation and Luteinization

JoAnne S. Richards, Jean Sirois, Usha Natraj,
Jacqueline K. Morris, Susan L. Fitzpatrick,
and Jeffrey W. Clemens

Two principal physiological events occur within preovulatory follicles as a consequence of the LH/FSH surge: ovulation and luteinization. The ovulation process culminates in the extrusion of the oocyte-cumulus complex and is dependent on a specific sequence of biochemical events. These biochemical changes include the rapid but transient increase in a novel, distinct isoform of *prostaglandin endoperoxide synthase* (PGS-2) (1–8), *tissue plasminogen activator* (tPA) (9, 10), and *progesterone receptor* (PR) (11–13). In contrast, luteinization is a process by which follicular granulosa and theca cells become nonmitotic and establish a specific, stable luteal cell phenotype. The biochemical changes that occur in response to the LH surge and are associated with luteinization include the marked and sustained induction of *cholesterol side-chain cleavage cytochrome P450* ($P450_{scc}$), as well as the dramatic and rapid decreases in mRNA for the *LH receptor* (LH-R), the regulatory *subunit β of type II cyclic AMP-dependent protein kinase* (RIIβ), aromatase, and 17α-hydroxylase ($P450_{17α}$) (Fig. 10.1) (14). Once luteinization has occurred, genes regulated by FSH/LH/cAMP in the follicle are no longer regulated by these agonists in the corpus luteum. This apparent transition from cAMP-dependent regulation to cAMP-independent regulation of these genes has prompted us to ask why surge (as opposed to basal) concentrations of LH are required to initiate these two diverse processes, what might be unique about the genes induced by the LH surge, and what intracellular signaling pathways might be involved.

It is well established that both FSH and LH bind to ligand-specific cell-surface receptors, leading to activation of adenylyl cyclase and cAMP production as well as to increases in intracellular calcium (15–21). Further-

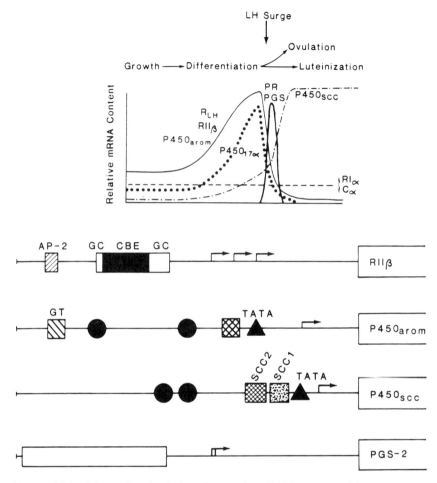

FIGURE 10.1. Schematic of relative changes in mRNA expressed in response to hormones during granulosa cell differentiation, ovulation, and luteinization. See text for discussion.

more, in rat preovulatory follicles the isoforms of protein kinase A that appear to be involved as a first step in transducing the cAMP signal are RIIβ and Cα (15, 16). Transcription factors known to be involved in cAMP regulation of specific genes in other tissues include AP-1 (Jun/Fos) (22, 23), CREB (22, 23), AP2 (24), and possibly steroid receptors (25). The role of any of these factors in regulating genes in the ovary is less well documented. Thus, other factors must be considered, identified, and characterized.

Evidence that cAMP plays a leading role in mediating the effects of low and ovulatory concentrations of gonadotropins in ovarian cell differentiation is well documented and hard to dispute (15, 16). For example, when granulosa cells obtained from small antral follicles are cultured in the presence of steroid (testosterone/estradiol) and either forskolin or FSH, they acquire a phenotype indistinguishable from that observed in granulosa cells of preovulatory follicles; for example, elevated levels of aromatase, LH-R, and RIIβ (16, 17, 26, 27). Furthermore, if these differentiated granulosa cells are then exposed to ovulatory concentrations of FSH or LH or high levels of forskolin, changes in gene expression mimic those observed in vivo as a consequence of the LH/FSH surge: induction of PGS-2 (6), PR (13), $P450_{scc}$ (28), and $\alpha_2$-macroglobulin (29) and suppression of aromatase, LH-R, and RIIβ (16, 17, 26, 27).

Despite the exhaustive litany supporting a primary role of cAMP mediating granulosa cell differentiation, there is also evidence that other pathways may be utilized. For example, gonadotropin receptors have been shown to be directly coupled to the phospholipase C-$Ca^{++}$-C-kinase pathway (20, 21). Thus, the differential effects of basal versus ovulatory levels of gonadotropins cannot be associated unequivocally with activation of either (or both) pathways. Furthermore, the promoters of genes expressed in granulosa cells in response to hormones exhibit markedly different structural features. Some of the genes (aromatase, $P450_{scc}$, and inhibin α) contain TATA and CAAT box motifs and initiate transcription at a single site (26–28, 30, 31). Other genes (PGS-2, PR, RIIβ, LH-R, and activin βB) lack TATA and CAAT box motifs and initiate transcription at multiple sites (32–38). Thus, although changes in mRNA for aromatase, RIIβ, and LH-R exhibit similar temporal changes in response to FSH and forskolin, the structure of their promoters differs markedly.

Of the genes described above, only inhibin α (31) contains a consensus *cAMP regulatory element* (CRE: TGACGTCA) to which the well-characterized CREB protein, as well as members of the CREB family (ΔCREB ATFs, C/EBP, and CREMs), binds (22, 23) and which is important for functional activity in granulosa cells in response to FSH/cAMP. Promoters of genes for aromatase and $P450_{scc}$ contain an AGGTCA motif that appears to confer hormone-tissue-specific inducibility in gonadal (aromatase and $P450_{scc}$) cells (30, 39) and adrenal ($P450_{scc}$) cells (40–42), yet the pattern of expression of these two genes in granulosa cells is markedly different. As noted, aromatase is induced by low but increasing levels of hormone and is turned off by the ovulatory hormone surge, whereas $P450_{scc}$ appears to require the LH surge for maximal induction and subsequent constitutive maintenance (26, 43, 44). Gel shift assays using aromatase and side-chain cleavage promoter sequences containing AGGTCA motifs indicate that the ability of nuclear proteins to bind this hexameric sequence is dependent on 5′ flanking, contexual sequences (30, 39, 42, 45). Thus, if the AGGTCA motif is involved in regulating the expression of each of these genes, one would predict that multiple factors are capable of binding this sequence and/or that transcription is regulated by differential modification (phosphorylation) of a limited number of factors.

Recent publications indicate that there are several proteins capable of binding the AGGTCA motif, that binding is dependent on contexual sequences, and that the proteins are present in a limited number of tissues (42, 44, 45). Furthermore, these proteins appear to belong to a subfamily of the orphan (steroid) receptor superfamily. Genes such as RIIβ, LH-R, PR, and activin βB have promoters that are highly GC rich (32–38), whereas the promoter for the novel, distinct isoform of PGS not only lacks the TATA-CAAT motifs, but also lacks GC-rich domains (preliminary data). Yet, the patterns of expression of PGS-2 (1–6) and PR (11–13) are highly similar. Both PGS-2 and PR mRNA and protein are rapidly but transiently induced by the LH/FSH surge—an effect that is restricted to differentiated granulosa cells possessing a preovulatory cell phenotype. Taken together, these observations suggest that sequences unique to genes turned on and transiently expressed (PGS-2 and PR) in response to the LH surge must be different from genes turned off by the LH surge (aromatase, LH-R, and RIIβ) or those turned on constitutively ($P450_{scc}$) (14). These different patterns suggest that these genes are not only expressed in a cell-specific manner in the ovary, but appear to be regulated by different *cis*-acting DNA motifs that recognize specific *trans*-acting factors. Thus, these DNA:protein regulatory units that do not appear to involve the CRE/CREB family need to be identified. Furthermore, the intracellular pathways leading to their activation/suppression need to be defined.

Evidence that pathways other than, or in addition to, the cAMP-A-kinase pathway are involved in gonadotropin action is indirect but, based on the foregoing discussion, requires special attention. First, it is known that GnRH (46, 47), as well as FSH and LH (15, 17), binds to ligand-specific receptors in rat granulosa cells and can induce ovulation (48, 49) in vitro. Second, GnRH, like FSH and LH at ovulatory concentrations, can induce the expression of enzymes presumed to play key roles in ovulation; namely, PGS-2 (1–6), PR (50), and tPA (9, 10). Third, GnRH induces these enzymes (mRNA and protein) without stimulating marked increases in cAMP or progesterone (5), thus suggesting that GnRH activates (shares) some, but not all, of the same pathways as elevated gonadotropins. Substantial evidence has accumulated to suggest that GnRH acts on pituitary gonadotropes primarily by increasing intracellular $Ca^{++}$ and protein kinase C. However, the restriction of GnRH action to the C-kinase pathway has been challenged (51).

Some of the inconsistencies in documenting an unequivocal role for C-kinase results from several factors. The GnRH receptor(s) has not yet been cloned. Furthermore, there are multiple forms of C-kinase, with varying requirements for $Ca^{++}$ and *diacyl glycerol* (DAG) as well as selective activation responses to phorbol esters. For example, *phorbol myristate acid* (PMA) will activate C-kinase α but not C-kinase βII, whereas bryostatin will selectively activate C-kinase βII (52). Thus, use of PMA as the sole indicator of C-kinase activity in cells does not necessarily mimic the complexity of the C-kinase signaling pathway and specific cellular responses to this pathway. Attempts to mimic the effects of GnRH on preovulatory follicles by substituting PMA or bryostatin have not been successful (5). Induction of PGS-2 was not observed in the presence of increasing doses of either C-kinase activator; nor did PMA/bryostatin cause the small increases in cAMP and progesterone observed when preovulatory follicles were incubated with GnRH. Furthermore, PMA alone is not able to induce luteinization. However, PMA has a small but demonstrable effect in cultured granulosa cells (Sirois and Richards, unpublished observations). Thus, any explanation of the effects of GnRH in ovarian function suffers from the same problems as mentioned above as well as its tissue specificity.

In addition, it is not known if the GnRH receptor in the ovary is the same as or different from that in the pituitary, despite similar binding affinities. Splice variants of receptors are common (35, 53, 54) and provide receptors with different intracellular, cytoplasmic domains such as that exhibited by the PRL receptor (55). Lastly, there is no solid evidence yet for an ovarian GnRH-like peptide that might be involved in the ovulatory process. Nonetheless, use of GnRH in the foregoing studies has provided an analytic way to compare and dissect what may be multiple pathways involved in cAMP action in the preovulatory follicle.

In addition to GnRH, *epidermal growth factor* (EGF), acting via the EGF receptor-associated tyrosine kinase, also induces PGS-2 (5) and tPA (10), albeit less effectively. That tyrosine kinases might be involved in mediating some of the actions of ovulatory doses of FSH/LH or GnRH has been supported by experiments using such tyrphostins as genistein (an ATP binding inhibitor) and AG18 (a substrate binding inhibitor) of tyrosine kinases (5, 56). Specifically, both of these tyrphostins block induction of PGS-2 by LH, FSH, forskolin, GnRH, and EGF (5 and preliminary results). Additionally, the induction of the chicken homolog of PGS-2 (CEF-147) (8) has been observed in chicken embryo fibroblasts transformed by the Rous sarcoma virus, thus implicating the tyrosine kinase $pp60^{v-src}$ as a potential regulator of this enzyme. Thus, one possible way to link the cAMP-A-kinase pathway with a tyrosine-kinase pathway in granulosa cells is to suggest that cAMP (at elevated concentrations) leads to the phosphorylation and activation of $pp60^{c-src}$. It is known that cAMP-A-kinase can activate $pp60^{c-src}$ in other systems (57).

*Acknowledgments.* Supported in part by NIH Grants HD-16229 and HD-16272 and fellowships to Jean Sirois (MRC), Susan L. Fitzpatrick (Laylor Foundation), and Jeffrey W. Clemens (NRSA).

## References

1. Hedin L, Gaddy-Kurten D, Kurten R, Richards JS. Prostaglandin endoperoxide synthase in rat ovarian follicles: content, cellular distribution, and evidence for hormonal induction preceding ovulation. Endocrinology 1987; 121:722–31.
2. Wong WYL, DeWitt DL, Smith WL, Richards JS. Rapid induction of prostaglandin endoperoxide synthase in rat preovulatory follicles by luteinizing hormone and cAMP is blocked by inhibitors of transcription and translation. Mol Endocrinol 1989;3:1714–23.
3. Wong WYL, Richards JS. Evidence for two antigenically distinct, molecular weight variants of prostaglandin H synthase in the rat ovary. Mol Endocrinol 1991;5:1269–79.
4. Sirois J, Richards JS. Identification and characterization of a novel distinct isoform of prostaglandin endoperoxide synthase. J Biol Chem 1991;267:6382–8.
5. Wong WYL, Richards JS. Induction of prostaglandin H synthase in rat preovulatory follicles by gonadotropin-releasing hormone. Endocrinology 1992;130:3512–21.
6. Sirois J, Simmons DL, Richards JS. Hormonal regulation of messenger ribonucleic acid encoding a novel isoform of prostaglandin endoperoxide H synthase in rat preovulatory follicles. J Biol Chem 1992;267:11586–92.
7. Kujubu D, Fletcher B, Varnam B, Lim R, Hershmann H. TIS 10, a phorbol ester tumor promoter-inducible mRNA from Swiss 3T3 cells, encodes a novel prostaglandin synthase/cyclo-oxygenase homologue. J Biol Chem 1991; 266:12866–72.
8. Xie W, Chapman JG, Robertson DL, Erickson RL, Simmons DL. Expression of a mitogen-responsive gene encoding prostaglandin synthase is regulated by mRNA splicing. Proc Natl Acad Sci USA 1991;88:2692–6.
9. Beers WH, Strickland S, Reich E. Ovarian plasminogen activator: relationship to ovulation and hormonal regulation. Cell 1975;6:387.
10. Galway AB, Oikawa M, Ny T, Hsueh AJW. Epidermal growth factor induction stimulates tissue plasminogen activator activity and messenger RNA levels in cultured rat granulosa cells: mediation by pathways independent of protein kinase-A and -C. Endocrinology 1989;125:126–35.
11. Park O-K, Mayo KE. Transient expression of progesterone receptor messenger RNA in ovarian granulosa cells after the preovulatory luteinizing hormone surge. Mol Endocrinol 1991;5:967–78.
12. Iwai M, Yasuda K, Fukuoka M, et al. Luteinizing hormone induces progesterone receptor gene expression in cultured porcine granulosa cells. Endocrinology 1991;129:1621–7.
13. Natraj U, Richards JS. Hormonal regulation of the progesterone receptor in cultured granulosa cells (in preparation).
14. Richards JS, Clemens JW, Sirois J, Fitzpatrick SL, Wong WYL, Kurten RC. Hormonal control of gene expression during ovarian cell differentiation. In: Leung PCK, Hsueh AJW, Friesen HG (eds), Molecular basis of reproductive endocrinology. New York: Springer-Verlag, 1993.
15. Richards JS. Maturation of ovarian follicles: actions and interactions of pituitary hormones on follicular cell differentiation. Physiol Rev 1980;60:51–89.

16. Richards JS, Jahnsen T, Hedin L, et al. Ovarian follicular development: from physiology to molecular biology. Recent Prog Horm Res 1987;43:231–76.
17. Segaloff DL, Wang H, Richards JS. Hormonal regulation of luteinizing hormone/chorionic gonadotropin receptor mRNA in rat ovarian cells during follicular development and luteinization. Mol Endocrinol 1990;4:1856–65.
18. Jonassen JA, Bose K, Richards JS. Enhancement and desensitization of hormone-responsive adenylyl cyclase in granulosa cells of preantral and antral ovarian follicles: effects of estradiol and FSH. Endocrinology 1982;111:74–9.
19. Hunzicker-Dunn M, Birnbaumer L. Adenylyl cyclase activities in ovarian tissues, III. Regulation of responsiveness to LH, FSH and $PGE_1$ in prepubertal, cycling, pregnant and pseudopregnant rats. Endocrinology 1976; 99:198–234.
20. Gudermann T, Birnbaumer M, Birnbaumer L. Evidence for dual coupling of the murine luteinizing hormone receptor to adenylyl cyclase and phosphoinositide breakdown and $Ca^{++}$ mobilization. J Biol Chem 1992;267:4479–88.
21. Davis JS, Weakland L, Farese R, West L. Luteinizing hormone increases inositol triphosphate and cytosolic free $Ca^{++}$ in isolated bovine luteal cells. J Biol Chem 1987;262:8515–21.
22. Roesler WJ, Vandenbark GR, Hanson RW. Cyclic AMP and the induction of eukaryotic gene expression. J Biol Chem 1988;263:9063–6.
23. Habener JF. Cyclic AMP response element binding proteins: a cornucopia of transcription factors. Mol Endocrinol 1990;4:1087–94.
24. Hyman SE, Comb M, Pearlberg J, Goodman HM. An AP-2 element acts synergistically with the cAMP and phorbol ester-inducible enhancer of the human proenkephalin gene. Mol Cell Biol 1989;9:321–4.
25. Evans RM. The steroid and thyroid hormone receptor superfamily. Science 1988;240:889–95.
26. Fitzpatrick SL, Richards JS. Regulation of cytochrome P450 aromatase mRNA and activity by steroids and gonadotropins in rat granulosa cells. Endocrinology 1991;129:1452–62.
27. Hickey GJ, Krasnow JS, Beattie WG, Richards JS. Aromatase cytochrome P450 in rat ovarian granulosa cells before and after luteinization: cAMP-dependent and independent regulation, cloning and sequencing of rat aromatase cDNA and 5′ genomic DNA. Mol Endocrinol 1990;4:3–12.
28. Oonk RB, Parker KL, Gibson JL, Richards JS. Rat cholesterol side-chain cleavage cytochrome P450 (P450scc) gene. Structure and regulation by cAMP in vitro. J Biol Chem 1990;265:22392–401.
29. Gaddy-Kurten D, Richards JS. Regulation of $\alpha_2$-macroglobulin by luteinizing hormone and prolactin during cell differentiation in the rat ovary. Mol Endocrinol 1991;5:1280–91.
30. Fitzpatrick SL, Richards JS. Characterization of the aromatase promoter (in preparation).
31. Pei L, Dodson R, Schoderbek WE, Maurer RA, Mayo KE. Regulation of the $\alpha$ inhibin gene by cyclic adenosine 3′,5′-monophosphate after transfection into rat granulosa cells. Mol Endocrinol 1991;5:521–34.
32. Sirois J, Richards JS. Characterization of the rat PGS-2 gene and its promoter (in preparation).
33. Kurten RC, Levy L, Shey J, Durica J, Richards JS. Identification and characterization of the GC-rich and cAMP-inducible promoter of the type IIβ

cAMP-dependent protein kinase regulatory subunit gene. Mol Endocrinol 1992;6:536–50.
34. Koo Y, Ji I, Slaughter RG, Ji TH. Structure of the luteinizing hormone receptor gene and multiple exons of the coding sequence. Endocrinology 1991;128:2297–308.
35. Tsai-Morris C, Buck OE, Wang W, Xie X, Dufau M. Structural organization of the rat luteinizing hormone (LH) receptor gene. J Biol Chem 1991; 266:11355–9.
36. Wang H, Nelson S, Ascoli M, Segaloff DL. The 5' flanking region of the rat lutropin/chorionic gonadotropin receptor gene confers Leydig cell expression and negative regulation of gene transcription by cAMP. Mol Endocrinol 1992;6:320–6.
37. Mason AJ, Berkemeier LM, Schmelzer CH, Schwall RH. Activin B: precursor sequences, genomic structures and in vitro activities. Mol Endocrinol 1989;3:1352–8.
38. Jeltsch J, Turcotte B, Garnier J, et al. Characterization of multiple mRNAs originating from the chicken progesterone receptor gene. J Biol Chem 1990;265:3967–74.
39. Clemens JW, Richards JS. (in preparation.)
40. Rice DA, Mouw AR, Bogerd AM, Parker KL. A shared promoter element regulates the expression of three steroidogenic enzymes. Mol Endocrinol 1991;5:1552–61.
41. Rice DA, Kirkman MS, Aitken LD, Mouw AR, Schimmer BP, Parker KL. Analysis of the promoter region of the gene encoding mouse cholesterol side-chain cleavage enzyme. J Biol Chem 1990;265:11713–20.
42. Lala DS, Rice DA, Parker KL. Steroidogenic factor 1, a key regulator of steroidogenic enzyme expression, is the mouse homolog of fushi tarazu-factor 1. Mol Endocrinol 1992;6.
43. Goldring NB, Durica JM, Lifka J, et al. Hormonal regulation of cholesterol side-chain cleavage P450 messenger RNA in rat ovarian follicles and constitutive expression in corpora lutea. Endocrinology 1987;120:1942–50.
44. Oonk RB, Krasnow JS, Beattie WG, Richards JS. Cyclic AMP-dependent and -independent regulation of cholesterol side-chain cleavage cytochrome P450 (P450scc) in rat ovarian granulosa cells and corpora lutea. J Biol Chem 1989;264:21934–42.
45. Wilson TE, Paulsen RE, Padgett KA, Milbrandt J. Participation of non-zinc finger residues in DNA binding by two nuclear orphan receptors. Science 1992;256:107 10.
46. Pieper D, Richards JS, Marshall J. Ovarian gonadotropin-releasing hormone (GnRH) receptors: characterization, distribution and induction by GnRH. Endocrinology 1981;108:1144–55.
47. Harwood JP, Clayton RN, Chen TC, Knox G, Catt KJ. Ovarian gonadotropin-releasing hormone receptors, II. Regulation and effects on ovarian development. Endocrinology 1980;107:414–21.
48. Koos RD, LeMaire WJ. The effects of a gonadotropin-releasing hormone agonist on ovulation and steroidogenesis during perfusion of rabbit and rat ovaries in vitro. Endocrinology 1985;116:628–32.
49. Ekholm C, Hillensjo T, Isaksson O. Gonadotropin-releasing hormone agonists stimulate oocyte meiosis and ovulation in hypophysectomized rats. Endocrinology 1981;108:2022–4.

50. Espey LL. Ovulation as an inflammatory reaction—a hypothesis. Biol Reprod 1980;22:73–106.
51. Conn PM. Does protein kinase C mediate pituitary actions of gonadotropin-releasing hormone? Mol Endocrinol 1989;3:755–7.
52. Hocevar BA, Fields AP. Selective translocation of βII-protein kinase C to the nucleus of human promyelocytic (HL60) leukemia cells. J Biol Chem 1991;266:28–33.
53. Segaloff DL, Sprengel R, Nikolics K, Ascoli M. The structure of the lutropin/chorionic gonadotropin receptor. Recent Prog Horm Res 1990;46:261–303.
54. Sprengel R, Braun T, Nikolics K, Segaloff DL, Seeburg PH. The testicular receptor for follicle stimulating hormone: structure and functional expression of the cloned cDNA. Mol Endocrinol 1990;4:525–30.
55. Shirota M, Banville D, Ali S, et al. Expression of two forms of prolactin receptor in rat ovary and liver. Mol Endocrinol 1990;4:1136–43.
56. Morris JL, Richards JS. (in preparation.)
57. Roach P. Multisite and hierarchal protein phosphorylation. J Biol Chem 1991;266:14139–42.

# 11
# Dynamics of Human Follicle Development

BART C.J.M. FAUSER, THIERRY D. PACHE, AND DICK C. SCHOOT

In 1979 the first report appeared on follicular growth during the normal menstrual cycle as determined by ultrasonography (1). Only cystic structures above 10 mm in size were regarded as follicles. During the days before the *luteinizing hormone* (LH) peak, follicle size and serum estradiol levels were strongly correlated. It was also noticed that growth of the follicle was linear, progressing 1.5–3 mm each day (2). Subsequently, numerous studies have focused on follicular growth and the diameter of the graafian follicle before disappearance (i.e., ovulation). Accuracy of sonographic estimates of follicle size was documented by comparison with the diameter derived from follicular volumes obtained during laparoscopic oocyte collection (3). Introduction of the transvaginal route was a major step toward better resolution (4, 5). Using this technique, follicles as small as 2 mm in diameter could be quantified reliably (6), which allows careful monitoring of the dynamics of development of dominant and nondominant follicles.

Data are accumulating underlining the significance of local (intraovarian) modification of gonadotropin action for regulation of gonadal function under normal, pathological, and pharmacological conditions. Awareness is growing that endocrine estimates in peripheral blood alone cannot explain all the conditions that clinicians are faced with. It appears that the classical concept of endocrine regulation of follicular development should be revised. In general, the stage of development of the follicle is represented by its size, which can be estimated by ultrasound. Follicle development is believed to be primarily regulated by *follicle stimulating hormone* (FSH) -induced granulosa cell aromatase activity. Regulation and function of these cells could be indicated by estimates in follicular fluid. It should therefore be possible to obtain additional information on the regulation of follicle development in the human by careful monitoring of intraovarian changes using transvaginal sonography and by correlating these observations with endocrine estimates in peripheral blood and follicular fluid. This chapter focuses on related studies performed by our group. Growth characteristics of ovarian follicles have been studied in regularly cycling controls, in women with cycle abnormalities, and during induction of ovulation with exogenous gonadotropins.

# Follicle Development During the Follicular Phase of the Normal Menstrual Cycle

Based on morphological studies by Gougeon and coworkers, it is believed that maturation of follicles from the primordial stage up to a graafian preovulatory follicle takes approximately 85 days. A cohort of follicles is stimulated for further synchronous development and gaining of gonadotropin dependence by the intercycle rise in FSH. This process is referred to as *recruitment* and may be viewed as a rescue of follicles from early atresia. Follicles reach the antral stage much earlier, at a size of ~0.2–0.3 mm, and can be observed by transvaginal sonography from a size of 2 mm. In vitro and in vivo data obtained so far in the human suggest that selection of the dominant follicle takes place around the midfollicular phase—presumably by the FSH enhancement of aromatase activity, allowing for dramatic increased production of estrogens—and the remaining follicles from the recruited cohort become atretic. In this way, development of a single dominant follicle is secured under normal conditions.

## *Selection and Growth of the Dominant Follicle*

Mechanisms underlying selection of the dominant follicle and subsequent monofollicular growth are largely unknown, but diminished stimulation of nondominant follicles by relatively low FSH levels in concert with intraovarian regulation might play an important role (7). Based on our own observations in 7 regularly cycling women (Fig. 11.1), it can be concluded that the presence of a dominant follicle can be ascertained on average 7 days before the LH surge (mean cycle day 8; Table 11.1) at a follicle diameter of 10 mm (6). Subsequent growth of the dominant follicle ranged between 1.4 and 2.2 mm/day, reaching a preovulatory size between 18 and 23 mm before ovulation (Fig. 11.2).

Our observations are in agreement with previous literature (for a comprehensive summary, see 8). Daily hormone estimates in peripheral blood in our control subjects showed that estradiol concentrations remain unchanged during the early follicular phase, with a rapid increase after formation of the dominant follicle (Fig. 11.3). Moreover, these data clearly show decreasing FSH concentrations during the follicular phase.

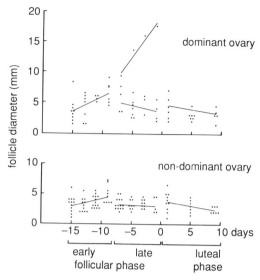

FIGURE 11.1. Diameter of individual follicles as measured by transvaginal sonography in one representative regularly cycling woman. Day 0 indicates the day of the LH surge. Indicated curves denote growth slopes (least-square regression lines) for dominant and nondominant follicles. Reprinted with permission from Pache, Wladimiroff, de Jong, Hop, and Fauser (6), © by The American Fertility Society.

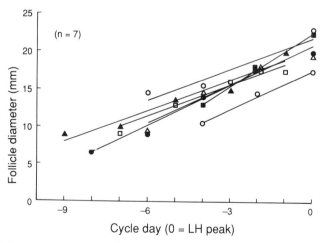

FIGURE 11.2. Growth rates of dominant follicles in 7 regularly cycling women. The number of observations per individual ranges between 3 and 5 (sonography performed every other day). Observed daily growth is between 1.4 and 2.2 mm. The size of the preovulatory follicle (calculated according to the day of the LH peak) is between 18.1 and 22.6 mm.

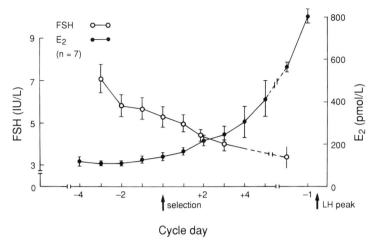

FIGURE 11.3. Daily FSH and estradiol serum levels in 7 regularly cycling women categorized according to the sonographic diagnosis of selection of the dominant follicle.

TABLE 11.1. Selection of the dominant follicle.

| Cycle characteristics | |
|---|---|
| Cycle length | 28.0 ± 1.9 days |
| Follicular phase length | 15.7 ± 1.6 days |
| Midluteal progesterone | 45.1 ± 4.9 nmol/L |
| Sonographic characteristics | |
| Presumed selection (cycle day) | 6.3 ± 2.3 |
| Size of selected follicle[a] | 9.9 ± 3.0 mm |

*Note:* Characteristics (mean ± SD) are based on sonographic criteria in 7 young, normal weight, regularly cycling women.
[a] Size from which a dominant follicle can be observed by transvaginal sonography.
*Source:* Based on data from Pache, Wladimiroff, de Jong, Hop, and Fauser (6).

These observations are in full agreement with classical endocrine literature, indicating that intrafollicular estrogen levels are high only in large follicles (9). Moreover, much higher estrogen concentrations were observed in venous blood draining an ovary bearing at least one large follicle (10).

## Growth of Nondominant Follicles

Monitoring the number and sizes of small, nondominant follicles could help to understand better the regulation of normal follicular development and polycystic transformation of ovaries in case of anovulation. Systemic evaluation of ovarian appearance under normal conditions could provide reference values for comparison with polycystic ovaries, ovaries under suppression by oral contraceptives or *gonadotropin releasing hormone* (GnRH) analogs, or under such stimulated conditions as during induction of ovulation or superovulation for in vitro fertilization.

In the early follicular phase, estrogen serum levels did not change (Fig. 11.3), and many small follicles could be observed by sonography. In our series the follicle number ranged between 6 and 8 per ovary. These follicles may represent atretic follicles from the previous cycle together with follicles that have been recruited for further development. Data on follicle size could not be analyzed longitudinally because individual nondominant follicles could not be identified in subsequent measurements. Growth slopes of the mean sizes of the observed cohort of nondominant follicles during successive days could be calculated, and a significant increase was observed for both ovaries in the early follicular phase (6). Growth slopes represent the net result of changes in the size of all individual follicles, a proportion of which will increase in size and a proportion of which will decrease in size.

## Follicle Maturation Arrest and Polycystic Ovaries

Ultrasonography represents a noninvasive technique to identify ovarian abnormalities in patients with *polycystic ovary syndrome* (PCOS). It seems important to focus on the ovary in these patients since anovulation and infertility are the most common complaints. Moreover, the success rates of induction of ovulation are reduced in these patients, and complication rates are augmented. At present, the sonographic picture of polycystic ovaries represents an important diagnostic feature for PCOS diagnosis. Enlarged ovaries were reported to be present in approximately 70% of patients with the clinical picture of PCOS, with cystic structures within the ovaries observed by transabdominal sonography in 30%–70% of cases (for review, see 11). Sonography may also enable one to determine both at what stage follicular maturation is arrested and how the sonographic appearance of ovaries relates to clinical and endocrine signs of PCOS and also to predict how ovaries will respond to induction of ovulation.

## Cessation of Follicle Maturation and Disturbed Selection in Polycystic Ovaries

It is generally believed that follicle maturation is arrested in PCOS due to disrupted FSH stimulation of granulosa cell aromatase activity (12). This defect can be overcome since follicle development does occur by elevating serum FSH levels following exogenous gonadotropin administration. Several lines of evidence indicate that cessation of development takes place at a stage where formation of the dominant follicle occurs under normal conditions. From a size of 10 mm, a single dominant follicle can be observed by transvaginal sonography (6). In polycystic ovaries the size of follicles rarely exceeds 8 mm in diameter (11, 13, 14). At this size intrafollicular estrogen production is stimulated under normal conditions (9, 10, 15, 16). Ongoing follicular development in the late follicular phase appears to be dependent on augmented intrafollicular estrogen production. However, no differences were observed between polycystic ovaries and nondominant follicles from normal ovaries when estradiol (or inhibin) and androstenedione levels were compared in fluid obtained from individual ovarian follicles (17).

This result is contradictory to several reports from the early 1960s (18) stating that estrogen levels were extremely low and that androgen concentrations were high. In these studies, pooled follicular fluid was used. We felt—considering potential changes in the follicular microenvironment—that fluid from individual follicles should be kept separate, and it was indeed confirmed that major differences among individuals preclude pooling (17). These observations are in favor of the concept of normal early follicular development and disturbed selection by absent local enhancement of the aromatase enzyme. It cannot be ruled out, however, that diminished secretion of other granulosa cell-derived factors, secreted concomitant with estrogens, is responsible for arrested follicle growth in PCOS. It is of interest to note that we have observed growth of ovarian follicles even with very low intrafollicular estrogen concentrations using recombinant human FSH in patients with isolated gonadotropin deficiency (16). The concept of disturbed selection is further supported by the observation that once formation of a single dominant follicle has taken place in PCOS patients during gonadotropin induction of ovulation, further development and serum estrogen levels are normal (19). Apparently, once selection has taken place in these patients by increased FSH stimulation, further development is indistinguishable from normal development.

## Differentiation Between Normal and Polycystic Ovaries by Transvaginal Sonography

Up until now, most studies related to the diagnosis of polycystic ovaries have been uncontrolled, using abdominal scanning, and were based mainly on the observed number of ovarian follicles. In some studies the diagnosis of PCOS has been based only on the presence of polycystic ovaries by sonography. In addition, polycystic ovaries have been reported to be present in a proportion of regularly cycling women.

In a controlled study using transvaginal sonography, it was recently shown (13) that discrimination by follicle number alone is difficult since a wide overlap was observed in the ovaries of regularly cycling women and the ovaries of PCOS patients. For instance, a threshold number of 10 follicles per ovary would yield a high specificity (we have never observed more than 10 follicles in normal ovaries) but low sensitivity (almost 50% of PCOS patients [diagnosis was based on endocrine criteria] exhibited less than 10 follicles per ovary). However, the use of additional sonographic criteria—such as ovarian volume, amount of stroma, and follicle size—could substantially improve the discriminating power (13).

## Ovarian Sonographic Changes and Endocrine and Clinical Signs of PCOS

In a large series of patients exhibiting polycystic ovaries, clinical signs of PCOS were found to be present in 60%–70% of cases, whereas endocrine signs could be found in only 40% of these patients (20). Since sonographic criteria for the diagnosis of polycystic ovaries are arbitrary, we have investigated ovarian polycystic changes in all women with cycle abnormalities and correlated these observations with clinical and endocrine signs of PCOS (13, 21). Significant correlations could be observed between follicle number and hirsutism (as estimated by the Ferriman and Galwey score), (immunoreactive and bioactive) LH concentrations, and serum T levels. Ovarian parameters did not correlate with body weight and correlated only partly with insulin resistance. These findings give further support to the notion that LH and androgens are involved in polycystic transformation of ovaries. It would be interesting to study whether the reduction of LH and T-levels by GnRH analog treatment would normalize the ovarian sonographic appearance. However, in patients with elevated immunoreactive LH concentrations and cycle abnormalities, the presence of polycystic ovaries is less frequent as compared to PCOS diagnosed on the basis of such clinical criteria as hirsutism and obesity (22).

## Follicle Development During Gonadotropin Stimulation of Ovarian Function

Major differences do exist between follicle development during the spontaneous menstrual cycle and follicle development during gonadotropin induction of ovulation. This may be partly due to the fact that mainly PCOS patients are involved. These patients are frequently resistant to clomiphene-citrate, and success rates during gonadotropin treatment are relatively poor, and complication rates are high (23). Moreover, the dose regimens used give rise to supraphysiological gonadotropin serum levels. As a consequence, the number of growing follicles is enhanced, and the process of selection of the dominant follicle is frequently disturbed, resulting in multiple follicular development. Therefore, in stimulated cycles the correlation between serum estrogen concentrations and follicle size is poor.

Sonography may be helpful for timing the *human chorionic gonadotropin* (hCG) injection to trigger ovulation in mature graafian follicles. In addition, development of the ovarian hyperstimulation syndrome—the most serious complication of gonadotropin treatment—can be predicted by the observed number of medium-sized follicles (24). The adjuvant use of serum estrogen concentrations may help to reduce further the incidence of ovarian hyperstimulation. At present, the low-dose, step-up dose regimen is widely used, starting with 1 amp/day for 1 or 2 weeks. Although results of this empirical treatment seem quite satisfactory (25), a physiological ground for this approach is lacking. The wide gap between ovulation and ongoing pregnancy rates indicates that other factors, such as oocyte quality, corpus luteum function, and endometrial receptivity, may be important additional factors for establishing a viable pregnancy.

## *Growth Patterns of Ovarian Follicles During Gonadotropin Treatment in PCOS Patients Using a Step-Down Dose Regimen*

In the late follicular phase, the dominant follicle continues to mature, even with clearly diminished FSH concentrations (see also, Figs. 11.2 and 11.3). Under normal conditions growth of the dominant follicle as compared to less-mature follicles appears to be less dependent on FSH, possibly because of the autocrine effects of high intrafollicular estrogen concentrations (26). Indeed, it was shown in the monkey that follicles can continue to mature in the presence of FSH concentrations that were unable to support growth of less-mature follicles (27). In addition, a step-down gonadotropin protocol showed better synchronization of follicle rupture, with reduced chances for delayed ovulations (28). It may therefore be hypothesized that incremental dose regimens unintentionally disturb the selection process and, therefore, provoke multiple follicular development.

Preliminary clinical observations suggest that the step-down dose regimen can be an alternative for induction of ovulation using exogenous gonadotropins (29). We have designed an initial study to investigate whether decreasing the gonadotropin dose (in combination with a GnRH analog to suppress endogenous pituitary gonadotropin secretion) after presumed selection would diminish the subsequent growth of nondominant follicles and still lead to ovulation (Fig. 11.4). Obtained data indicate that ovulation can be induced using this dose regimen. Observed reduced numbers of medium-sized follicles, together with a decrease in serum estrogen levels, indicate that these follicles are functionally active (30). At present, we are testing the clinical relevance of these initial observations by adjusting the decremental dose regimen and using different preparations (including purified FSH) in a larger-population patient series (Schoot et al. and Donderwinkel et al., unpublished observations).

## Human Recombinant FSH in a Hypogonadotropic Woman: Estrogens and Follicle Development

Based on studies in animal species, it is generally believed that estrogens are essential for normal follicular development (26). Recent clinical observations have challenged the significance of this concept for the human (31, 32). Our participation in a multicenter study on safety and pharmacokinetic characteristics of human recombinant FSH in hypogonadotropic subjects provided the unique opportunity to evaluate whether LH is mandatory for normal estrogen production and subsequent follicle development. It was observed that follicle growth can be stimulated up to a preovulatory size with very low estrogen serum levels comparable to early follicular-phase levels. Follicular fluid estrogen concentrations in these graafian follicles were extremely low as compared to normal (16) and in the same order of magnitude as observed in small, nondominant follicles (17). These data indicate that the two-cell, two-gonadotropin hypothesis is operative in the human and that—next to FSH—sufficient amounts of LH are important for normal estrogen production by ovarian follicles. Since growth of preovulatory follicles can be induced with only FSH, it should be questioned whether estrogen biosynthesis is required for normal follicular development.

# Relevance of Monitoring Ovarian Function Under Other Clinical Conditions

## Controlled Ovarian Hyperstimulation and In Vitro Fertilization

The IVF procedure was introduced in a spontaneous cycle with laparoscopic aspiration of a single follicle. Shortly thereafter, it was demonstrated that the success rate of IVF was proportional to the number of transferred embryos. Numerous stimulation regimens developed for the

11. Dynamics of Human Follicle Development    143

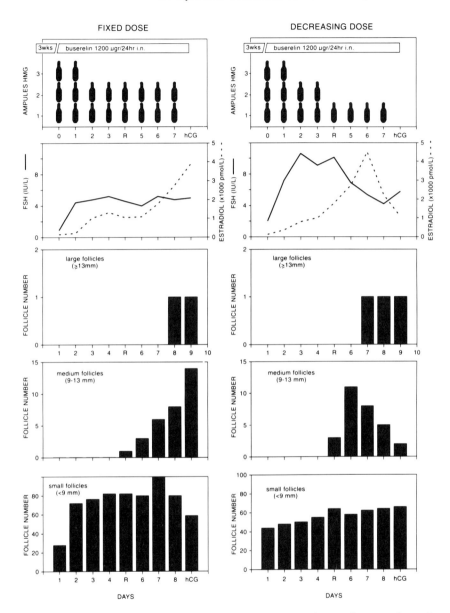

FIGURE 11.4. Schematic representation of 2 tested regimens for gonadotropin induction of ovulation with adjuvant GnRH analog treatment. The fixed-dose regimen included similar HMG doses following selection of the dominant follicle (left panel), whereas in the decreasing-dose regimen (right panel), medication was reduced to 1 amp/day (=75 IU) IM. Declining serum FSH concentrations in the latter group were followed by decreases in the number of medium-sized (between 9 and 13 mm) follicles and reduced estrogen outputs.

induction of multiple follicle development have been introduced (33, 34). Although serum estrogen levels are very high before the puncture of multiple follicles, the incidence of ovarian hyperstimulation is relatively low (35). This may be due to the aspiration of follicular fluid and granulosa cells, which subsequently reduces the amount of steroid-producing cells in the luteal phase. Therefore, the predictive value of follicle number before hCG administration for the occurrence of ovarian hyperstimulation is much less for IVF as compared to gonadotropin induction of ovulation. The amount of developing follicles can be monitored during "controlled" hyperstimulation, and sonography is a helpful tool for timing of the administration of hCG and for oocyte retrieval. Ovarian response during various stimulation regimens appears to be of limited significance for IVF outcome. The observed discrepancy between fertilization rates (80%–90%) and pregnancy rates (~20%) has focused attention on oocyte quality, the luteal phase, and endometrial function during IVF cycles.

## Follicular Development During Combined Oral Contraceptives

Recruitment, resulting in the synchronous growth of a cohort of follicles, is believed to be initiated by the intercycle rise in FSH. Under normal conditions, around the midfollicular phase at a size of 10 mm, a dominant follicle is selected for further development. During combined oral contraceptive medication, at the end of the 7-day, pill-free interval, gonadotropin serum levels are indistinguishable from the normal follicular phase, although estrogen levels are somewhat lower (36).

It is quite likely that follicle recruitment has already been initiated before contraceptive medication of the following month is started. Indeed, ovarian follicles above 10 mm in size have been observed in roughly 30% of women using oral contraceptives (37–39). By extending the pill-free interval, it was shown that these follicles have the capacity for continuous growth and subsequent rupture (40). Apparently, ongoing follicle maturation is arrested at a stage just before selection of the dominant follicle takes place under normal conditions by suppressing FSH levels below the threshold for further follicular development. FSH suppression is caused by the commencement of contraceptive medication after the pill-free interval, and it has been suggested that a 7-day, pill-free interval should be considered the maximum permitted.

The frequent occurrence of polycystic-like sonographic ovarian changes in women using oral contraceptives (39) may further indicate that absent formation of the dominant follicle may also affect the process of atresia of the remaining follicles from the recruited cohort. This may represent a situation similar to follicle maturation arrest and the augmented total number of follicles in polycystic ovaries.

## Conclusions

The significance of local modification of gonadotropin action for regulation of gonadal function under normal and pathophysiological conditions has been emphasized by numerous in vitro and in vivo observations. In the human, careful monitoring of intraovarian changes as assessed by transvaginal ultrasonography and hormone estimates in follicular fluid has proven to give additional information helpful for understanding the regulation of follicular development under various clinical circumstances. So far, these conditions mainly involve etiology and diagnosis of disturbed ovarian function and treatment of anovulation using exogenous gonadotropins in PCOS patients. It might be speculated that more insight into the suppressive activity of various oral contraceptive regimens might also help us to understand better the efficacy aspects of contraceptive medication.

*Acknowledgments.* The continuous support of Dr. J. Wladimiroff (Department of Obstetrics and Gynecology, Dijkzigt University Hospital) and Dr. F.H. de Jong (Department of Medicine III, Dijkzigt University Hospital) is highly appreciated.

## *References*

1. Hackeloer BJ, Fleming R, Robinson HP, Adam AH, Coutts JRT. Correlation of ultrasonic and endocrinologic assessment of human follicular development. Am J Obstet Gynecol 1979;135:122-8.
2. Renaud RL, Macler J, Dervain I, et al. Echographic study of follicular maturation and ovulation during the normal menstrual cycle. Fertil Steril 1980;33:272-6.
3. Leerentveld RA, van Gent I, vd Stoep M, Alberda ATh, Wladimiroff JW. Comparison of graafian follicle dimensions as determined by static and real-time sector scanning. Fertil Steril 1984;42:292-331.
4. Coleman BC, Arger PH, Grumbach K. Transvaginal and transabdominal sonography: prospective comparison. Radiology 1988;168:639-43.
5. Nyberg DA. Ultrasonography in reproductive endocrinology and infertility. In: Soules MR, ed. Current topics in obstetrics and gynecology: controversies in reproductive endocrinology and infertility. New York: Elsevier, 1989: 229-70.
6. Pache TD, Wladimiroff JW, de Jong FH, Hop WCJ, Fauser BCJM. Growth patterns of nondominant ovarian follicles during the normal menstrual cycle. Fertil Steril 1990;54:638-44.
7. Hodgen GD. The dominant follicle. Fertil Steril 1982;38:281-300.
8. Nitschke-Dabelstein S. Monitoring of follicular development using ultrasonography. In: Insler V, Lunenfeld B, eds. Infertility: male and female. Edinburgh: Livingston, 1986:101-25.
9. Hillier SG, vdBoogaard AMJ, Reichert LE, vHall EV. Intraovarian sex steroid hormone interactions and the regulation of follicle maturation: aroma-

tization of androgens by human granulosa cells in vitro. J Clin Endocrinol Metab 1980;50:640–5.
10. Baird DT, Fraser IS. Concentration of estrone and estradiol in follicular fluid and ovarian venous blood of women. Clin Endocrinol (Oxf) 1975;4:259–66.
11. Fauser BCJM. Classification of chronic hyperandrogenic anovulation. In: Coelingh-Bennink HJT, Vemer HM, v Keep PA, eds. Chronic hyperandrogenic anovulation. Park Ridge, NJ: Parthenon, 1991:13–17.
12. Yen SSC. The polycystic ovary syndrome. Clin Endocrinol (Oxf) 1980;12:177–208.
13. Pache TD, Hop WCJ, Wladimiroff JW, Schipper J, Fauser BCJM. Transvaginal sonography and abnormal ovarian appearance in menstrual cycle disturbances. Ultrasound Med Biol 1991;17:589–93.
14. Pache TD, Wladimiroff JW, Hop WCJ, Fauser BCJM. How to discriminate between normal and polycystic ovaries. Radiology 1992;183:421–3.
15. Erickson GF, Hsueh AJW, Quiqley ME, Rebar RW, Yen SSC. Functional studies of aromatase activity in human granulosa cells from normal and polycystic ovaries. J Clin Endocrinol Metab 1979;49:514–9.
16. Schoot DC, Coelingh-Bennink HJT, Mannaerts BMJL, Lamberts SWJ, Bouchard Ph, Fauser BCJM. Human recombinant FSH induces growth of preovulatory follicles without concomitant increase in androgen and estrogen biosynthesis in a woman with isolated gonadotropin deficiency. J Clin Endocrinol Metab 1992;74:1471–3.
17. Pache TD, Hop WCJ, de Jong FH, et al. Oestradiol, androstenedione, and inhibin levels in fluid from individual follicles of normal and polycystic ovaries, and in ovaries from androgen-treated female to male transsexuals. Clin Endocrinol (Oxf) 1992;36:565–71.
18. Axelrod LR, Goldzieher JW. The polycystic ovary, III. Steroid biosynthesis in normal and polycystic ovarian tissue. J Clin Endocrinol Metab 1962;22:431–40.
19. Schoot DC, Hop WCJ, Pache TD, de Jong FH, Fauser BCHM. Growth of the dominant follicle in spontaneous cycles and gonadotropin-stimulated polycystic ovary syndrome patients (submitted).
20. Conway GS, Honour LW, Jacobs HS. Heterogeneity of the polycystic ovary syndrome: clinical, endocrine and ultrasound features in 556 patients. Clin Endocrinol (Oxf) 1989;30:459–70.
21. Pache TD, de Jong FH, Hop WCJ, Fauser BCJM. Association between ovarian changes assessed by transvaginal sonography and clinical and endocrine signs of the polycystic ovary syndrome (submitted).
22. Fauser BCJM, Pache TD, Hop WCJ, de Jong FH, Dahl KD. Significance of serum LH measurements in women with cycle disturbances: discrepancies between immunoreactive and bioactive hormone estimates. Clin Endocrinol (Oxf) 1992.
23. Diamond MP, Wentz AC. Ovulation induction with human menopausal gonadotropins. Obstet Gynecol Surv 1986;41:480–9.
24. Blankstein J, Shalev J, Saadon T, et al. Ovarian hyperstimulation syndrome: prediction by number and size of preovulatory ovarian follicles. Fertil Steril 1987;47:597–602.
25. Hamilton-Fairley D, Kiddy D, Watson H, Sagle M, Franks S. Low-dose gonadotropin therapy for induction of ovulation in 100 women with polycystic ovary syndrome. Hum Reprod 1991;6:1095–9.

26. Hsueh AJW. Paracrine mechanisms involved in granulosa cell differentiation. Clin Endocrinol Metab 1986;15:117–34.
27. Zeleznik AJ, Kubik CJ. Ovarian response in macaques to pulsatile infusion of FSH and LH: increased sensitivity of the maturing follicle to FSH. Endocrinology 1986;119:2025–32.
28. Abbashi R, Kenigsberg D, Danforth D, Falk RJ, Hodgen GD. Cumulative ovulation rate in HMG/HCG treated monkeys: step-up versus step-down dose regimens. Fertil Steril 1987;47:1019–24.
29. Mizunuma H, Takagi T, Yamada K, Andoh K, Ibuki Y, Igarashi M. Ovulation induction by step down administration of purified urinary FSH in patients with polycystic ovary syndrome. Fertil Steril 1991;55:1195–6.
30. Schoot DC, Pache TD, Hop WC, de Jong FH, Fauser BCJM. Growth patterns of ovarian follicles during induction of ovulation with decreasing doses of HMG following presumed selection in polycystic ovary syndrome. Fertil Steril 1992;57:1117–20.
31. Rabinovici J, Blankstein J, Goldman B, et al. In vitro fertilization and primary embryonic cleavage are possible in 17α-hydroxylase deficiency despite extremely low intrafollicular 17β-estradiol. J Clin Endocrinol Metab 1991;68:693–7.
32. Chappel SC, Howles C. Reevaluation of the roles of LH and FSH in the ovulatory process. Hum Reprod 1991;9:1206–12.
33. Meldrum DR. Ovulation induction for in vitro fertilization procedures. Sem Reprod Endocrinol 1990;8:213–8.
34. Oehinger S, Hodgen GD. Induction of ovulation for assisted reproduction programmes. Baillieres Clin Obstet Gynaecol 1990;4:541–73.
35. Golan A, Ron-El R, Herman A, Soffer Y, Weinraub Z, Caspi E. Ovarian hyperstimulation syndrome: an update review. Obstet Gynecol Surv 1989;44:430–40.
36. vdSpuy ZM, Sohnius U, Pienaar CA, Schall R. Gonadotropin and estradiol secretion during the week of placebo therapy in oral contraceptive pill users. Contraception 1990;42:597–609.
37. Hamilton CJCM, Hoogland HJ. Longitudinal ultrasonographic study of the ovarian suppressive activity of a low-dose triphasic oral contraceptive during correct and incorrect pill intake. Am J Obstet Gynecol 1989;161:1159–62.
38. Thomas K, Vankrieken L. Inhibition of ovulation by low-dose monophasic contraceptive containing gestodene. Am J Obstet Gynecol 1990;163:1404–10.
39. Tayob Y, Robinson G, Adams J, et al. Ultrasound appearance of the ovaries during the pill-free interval. Br J Fam Plan 1990;16:94–6.
40. Killick SR. Ovarian follicles during oral contraceptive cycles: their potential for ovulation. Fertil Steril 1989;52:580–2.

# Part III
Intraovarian Regulatory Systems

# 12

# Structural and Functional Studies of Insulin-Like Growth Factor Binding Proteins in the Ovary

N.C. LING, X.-J. LIU, M. MALKOWSKI, Y.-L. GUO, G.F. ERICKSON, AND S. SHIMASAKI

During each estrous cycle, only a limited number of recruited follicles in the mammalian ovary will undergo the complete process of growth and development, ending in ovulation and corpus luteum formation, while the remainder succumb to degenerative atresia (1). Although it is well known that the primary regulators of the estrous cycle are the pituitary gonadotropins, FSH and LH, the detailed mechanisms regulating folliculogenesis are not well understood (2, 3). Among its numerous actions in the ovary, one of the critical functions of FSH is to stimulate the granulosa cells in the developing follicles to proliferate and produce estradiol, the steroid thought to be important for follicle maturation (4). To account for the development of selected follicles, it has been postulated that the follicular fluid in the antrum of the growing follicles contains polypeptides that block the action of FSH either by inhibiting the binding of FSH to its receptor at the cell membrane (5) or by blocking the postreceptor events induced by the binding of FSH (6) and thus causing follicle atresia. Since follicle survival and atresia are the very essence of propagation and preservation of the species, it is crucial to understand the regulatory mechanisms by which a cohort of recruited developing follicles branch away in two directions; that is, to continue growth or succumb to atresia. Therefore, we initiated a project in 1988 to isolate and identify the FSH-action inhibitors present in ovarian follicular fluid.

## Isolation and Characterization of an FSH-Action Inhibitor in Ovarian Follicular Fluid

Using a well-defined rat granulosa cell culture bioassay (7) that quantitates the effect of FSH on estradiol production to monitor the purification, a polypeptide was isolated from follicular fluid of the porcine ovary that specifically inhibited the FSH-stimulated production of estradiol (8). The purification scheme employed involved precipitation of the high molecular weight proteins in the follicular fluid with ammonium sulfate, followed by dialysis of the supernatant in 30% (vol/vol) acetic acid, gel filtration chromatography of the dialyzed material in Sephacryl S-200 superfine under acidic conditions, and several steps of reversed-phase HPLC. Microsequence analysis of the purified inhibitor, however, revealed that its sequence was very similar to the aminoterminal amino acid sequence of a recently characterized 53-kd growth hormone-dependent insulin-like growth factor binding protein from human serum (9), later designated as IGFBP-3 (10). Therefore, the FSH-action inhibitor isolated from ovarian follicular fluid could be the porcine cognate of the human IGFBP-3.

In order to ascertain this finding, we immediately screened porcine ovarian and liver cDNA libraries with a synthetic oligonucleotide probe based on an internal amino acid sequence derived from trypsin digestion of the inhibitor and cloned its cDNA (11). The deduced amino acid sequence of the cDNA confirmed that the purified inhibitor was indeed the porcine IGFBP-3.

## Identification of Five IGFBPs in Porcine Follicular Fluid and Adult Rat Serum

There is now substantial evidence for autocrine and paracrine actions of IGF-I in the ovary (12). Immunoreactive IGF-I is secreted by cultured granulosa cells (13), and its mRNA was detected by in situ hybridization to the granulosa cells of healthy follicles (14, 15). In rat granulosa cells cultured in serum-free medium, IGF-I acts synergistically with FSH to stimulate the production of estradiol (16), progesterone (17), LH receptor (18), inhibin (19), and follistatin (20, 21). Likewise, IGF-I acts synergistically with LH to stimulate androgen production by purified rat thecal and secondary interstitial cells cultured in serum-free medium (22–24). Moreover, IGF-I receptors have been located by binding experiments (25, 26) and in situ hybridization studies (27, 28) on the thecal and granulosa cells. Thus, the inhibitory effect exerted by the purified IGFBP-3 could be due to sequestration of the endogenously produced IGF-I by the exogenous BP (29).

At the time when we identified IGFBP-3 as the FSH-action inhibitor in porcine ovarian follicular fluid, two other IGFBPs, designated IGFBP-1 (30–34) and IGFBP-2 (35–37), had already been characterized. Moreover, IGFBP-1 had been detected in human follicular fluid by RIA (38). However, it was not certain whether IGFBP-1 and IGFBP-2 were also present in porcine follicular fluid or if additional, unknown IGFBPs could

12. Insulin-Like Growth Factor Binding Proteins in the Ovary

be found in the ovary. To fully comprehend the physiological roles played by the various IGFBPs in the ovary, we undertook a comprehensive purification scheme to isolate and identify all IGFBPs present in porcine follicular fluid.

The IGFBPs were isolated by gel filtration chromatography, followed by affinity chromatography and several steps of reversed-phase HPLC (39). The gel filtration step was carried out under acidic medium to dissociate and separate the endogenous IGFs from their BPs in the follicular fluid. All the IGFBP-containing fractions from the gel filtration column were pooled and, after dialysis in phosphate-buffered saline at pH 7.4, selectively concentrated on an IGF-II-coupled Affi-Gel 15 column; the recovered material was further fractionated by reversed-phase HPLC. The purified HPLC peaks were subjected to amino acid sequence analysis. Table 12.1 shows the results of microsequence analysis of the aminoterminal amino acid sequence of the HPLC-purified IGFBPs. Peaks I, IIb, and IIIb have an aminoterminal amino acid sequence identical to that of porcine IGFBP-3. Peaks VIb and VII corresponded to the aminoterminal amino acid sequence of rat and human IGFBP-2. Peaks IIa and IIIa contained an identical but unknown amino acid sequence that was later designated IGFBP-5 (40). Peaks IVa and Va revealed an identical but novel amino acid sequence that was later designated IGFBP-6 (40). Peaks IVb and VIa showed an identical amino acid sequence that had not been reported before. This protein was later designated IGFBP-4 (40).

From this thorough analysis of the IGFBPs in porcine follicular fluid, two known IGFBPs, BP-2 and BP-3, plus three novel IGFBPs, BP-4, BP-5 and BP-6, were isolated. IGFBP-1 was not isolated under our experimental conditions.

TABLE 12.1. Aminoterminal amino acid sequences of porcine follicular fluid IGFBPs.

| HPLC peaks | | Amino acid sequence |
| --- | --- | --- |
| I | (BP-3) | G S G A V G T G P V |
| IIa | (BP-5) | L G S F V H X E P X D E K A L |
| IIb | (BP-3) | G S G A V G T G P V V R X E P X D |
| IIIa | (BP-5) | L G S F V H X E P X D E K A L S M X P P |
| IIIb | (BP-3) | G S G A V G T G P V V |
| IVa | (BP-6) | A Q X P G X G Q G V Q T G X P G |
| IVb | (BP-4) | D E A I H X P P X S E E K L A R X R P P V G |
| Va | (BP-6) | A Q X P G X G Q G |
| VIa | (BP-4) | D E A I H X P P X S E E K L A R X R P |
| VIb | (BP-2) | F R X P P X T P E S L A A X R P P P A A P P |
| VII | (BP-2) | F R X P P X T P E S |

*Note:* The amino acids are shown in one-letter code, and the sequences were determined by an ABI 470A protein sequenator. (X = a residue [probably cysteine] that was not identified.)

Since the animal model that we employed to study folliculogenesis was the rat, we needed to determine whether the same number of distinct IGFBPs was also present in the rat species. Also, because it is impossible to obtain a large volume of rat ovarian follicular fluid, we resorted to adult rat serum to isolate all of the IGFBPs. Using the same purification methodology, five IGFBPs corresponding to IGFBP-2, -3, -4, -5, and -6 were isolated from adult rat serum (41), as shown in Table 12.2. Again, IGFBP-1 was not found by our purification method. Because the complete primary structures of IGFBP-6, -5, and -4 were not known prior to our study, we immediately proceeded to clone their cDNAs from rat ovarian and human placental libraries (39, 41, 42).

## Amino Acid Sequence Comparison of Six IGFBPs

Figure 12.1 shows the most favorable alignment of the deduced amino acid sequences from the cDNAs of the novel IGFBP-4, -5, and -6, together with the previously characterized IGFBP-1, -2 and -3 in the rat and human species. None of the IGFBPs bears any amino acid sequence homology to the type I or type II IGF receptors. The homologous amino acid sequence regions among these six IGFBPs are located at the aminoterminal third and carboxyterminal third of the molecules, while the middle portion of the molecules is the most divergent.

There are 18 cysteines in rat and in human IGFBP-1, -2, -3, and -5, and their locations in the molecules are totally conserved. Among those 18

TABLE 12.2. Aminoterminal amino acid sequences of adult rat serum IGFBPs.

| HPLC peaks | | Amino acid sequence | |
|---|---|---|---|
| I | (BP-3) | GAGAVGAGPVVRXEPXD | |
| IIa | (BP-5) | LGSFVHXEPXDEKALSM | (major sequence) |
| | (BP-3) | GAGAVGAG | (minor sequence) |
| IIb | (BP-3) | GAGAVGAGPV | |
| IIIa | (BP-5) | LGSFVHXEPXDEKALSMXPPSPLGXELVKEPGXGXX | (major sequence) |
| | (BP-3) | GAGAVGAGPVVR | (minor sequence) |
| IIIb | (BP-3) | GAGAVGAGPVVRXEPXDARA | (major sequence) |
| | (BP-3) | KVDYESQSTD | (minor sequence) |
| | (BP-3) | YESQSTD | (minor sequence) |
| IVa | (BP-5) | LGSFVHXEPXDEKALSMXPPS | |
| IVb | (BP-3) | GAGAVGAGPVVRXEPXDARA | |
| V | (BP-4) | DEAIHXPPXSEEKLARXRP | (major sequence) |
| | (BP-6) | ALAGXPGXGPGVQ | (minor sequence) |
| VI | (BP-2) | EVLFRXPPXTPERLAAXGPPPDA | (major sequence) |
| | (BP-4) | DEAIHXPPXSEE | (minor sequence) |

*Note:* The amino acids are shown in one-letter code, and the sequences were determined by an ABI 470A protein sequenator. (X = a residue [probably cysteine] that was not identified.) In some peaks more than one amino acid sequence was detected, and they were designated as major and minor sequences.

cysteines, 12 are located at the aminoterminal of the molecule, spanning the first third of the total amino acid sequence, and the remaining 6 lie in the carboxyterminal region, spanning the last third of the protein sequence. IGFBP-4 contains 2 extra cysteines at the midregion of the molecule in addition to the 18 conserved cysteines. By contrast, rat IGFBP-6 and human IGFBP-6 contain only 14 and 16 cysteines, respectively. Eight of the 14 cysteines in the rat protein are located at the aminoterminal region of the molecule, whereas the human homolog contains 10 cysteines in the same region. The carboxyterminal region of both rat and human IGFBP-6 contains the remaining 6 conserved cysteines.

The absence of 4 and 2 cysteines in the rat and human IGFBP-6 amino acid sequences, respectively, resulted in the loss of the invariant Gly-Cys-Gly-Cys-Cys sequence present in all of the other five IGFBPs. Human IGFBP-3 and rat IGFBP-3 contain 3 and 4 potential Asn-linked glycosylation sites, respectively, and both human and rat IGFBP-4 possess 1 potential Asn-linked glycosylation site in the midregion of the molecule. Only human, but not rat, IGFBP-6 has a potential Asn-linked glycosylation site at the extreme carboxyterminal of the molecule.

## Localization of IGFBP mRNAs in the Rat Ovary

Northern analysis of the six IGFBP mRNAs in random cycling adult rat ovaries revealed mRNA transcripts of 1.8, 2.6, 2.6, 6.0, and 1.3 kb for IGFBP-2, -3, -4, -5, and -6, respectively. IGFBP-1 mRNA was not detectable (43). Using in situ hybridization, the cellular localization of IGFBP mRNAs was examined in adult rat ovaries, and the results are shown in Table 12.3 (p. 158). IGFBP-2 mRNA was localized specifically in thecal interstitial cells and secondary interstitial cells of the ovary (43). The IGFBP-2 transcript was very strong in thecal interstitial cells of secondary, tertiary, and graafian follicles (healthy and atretic); very strong in all secondary interstitial cells located in different regions of the ovary; and weak in thecal interstitial cells of preantral follicles. Surface epithelial cells also showed a positive signal for IGFBP-2. The IGFBP-3 hybridization signal was localized specifically to some corpora lutea. Here, the hybridization signal for IGFBP-3 was strong and distributed throughout the corpus luteum, strong but localized to only some luteal cells, or not detectable.

The IGFBP-4 mRNA was localized almost exclusively to granulosa cells of atretic follicles and was especially strong in those with a large antrum (atretic graafian follicles). Morphologically, the outer layer of granulosa cells was positive, while cells in the cumulus oophorus were negative. In some cases, IGFBP-4 signals were detected in the thecal interstitial cells, but they were weak and variable. The IGFBP-5 transcript was expressed in granulosa cells of atretic follicles and was especially

```
                              *              *           *        *    ***                 *                    *
Rat IGFBP-1                                         APCPWHCAPCTAERLELCPPVP-AS-CPEISRPAGCGCCPTCALPLGAACCVATAACAQGLSCRALPGEPRPLHALTRGQGAC
Rat IGFBP-2                                              EVLFRCPPCTPERLAACGPPPDAP-CAELVREPGCGCCSVCARQEGEACGVYIPRCAQTLRCYNPGSELPLKALVTGAGTC
Rat IGFBP-3                                   GAGAVGAGPVVRCEPCDARALAQCAPPPTAPACTELVREPGCGCCLTCALREGDACGVYTERCGTLRCQPRPAEQYPLKALLNGRGFC
Rat IGFBP-4                                              DEAIHCPPCSEEKLARCRPPVG---CEELVREPGCGCCATCALGLGMPCGVYTPRCGSGMRCYPPRGVEKPLRTLMHGQGVC
Rat IGFBP-5                                              LGSFVHCEPCDEKALSMC-PPSP-LGC-ELVKEPGCGCCMTCALAEGQSCGVYTERCAQGLRCLPRQDEEKPLHALLHGRGVC
Rat IGFBP-6                                                ALAGCPGC----(GPGVQEEDAGSPAD)----GCAETGCFRREGQPCGVYIPKCAPGLQCQPRENEETPLRALLIGQGRC

(VLEPPPATSSLSGSQHEEAKAAVASEDELAESPEMTEQLLDSFHLMAPSREDQPILWNAISTYSSMRAREITDLKKWE)
(EKRRVGATPQQVADSEDDHSEGGLIVENHVDGTMNMLGGSSAGRKPPKSGMKELAVFREKVNEQHRQMGKGAKHLSLEEPKKLRPPPART)
(ANASAASNLSAYLPSQPSPGNTESEEDHNAGSVESQVVPSTHRVIDSKFHPLHSKMEVIIKQARDSQRYKVDYESQSTDTQNFSESKRETEYG)
(TELSIEAIQESLQTSDKDESEHPNNSFNPCSAHDHRCLQKHMAKVRDRSKMKVVGTPREEPRPVPQG)
(LNEKSYGEQTKIERDSREHEEPTSEMAEEYSPKVFRFKHTRISELKAEAVKKDFRKKLTQSKFVGGAENTAHPRVIPAPEMRQESDG)
(QRARGPSEETTKESKPHGGASRPRDRDRQKNPRTSAAPIRPSPVQDGEMG)

 *                                     *                      *                    *
PCQRELYKVLERLAAQQKA--GD-E--IYKFYLPNCNKNGFYHSKQCETSLDGEAGLCWCVPWSGKKIPGSLETRGDPNCHQYFNVQN                        247 AA    Calc. MW
PCQQELDQVLERISTMRLPDDRGPLEHLYSLHIPNCDKHGLYNLKQCKMSLNGQRGECWCVNPTGKPIQAPTIRGDPECHLFYNEQQENDGVHAQRVQ              270 AA    26.8 kDa
PCRREMEDTLNHLKFLNVLSPRGV---HIPNCDKKGFYKKKQCRPSKGRKRGFCWCVDKYGQPLPGYDTKGKDDVHCLSVQSQ                             265 AA    29.6 kDa
SCQSELHRALERLAASQ--S-RTH-EDLFIIPIPNCDRNGNFHPRKCHPALDGORGFCWCVDRKTGVKLPGGLEPKGELDCQLADSLQE                       233 AA    28.9 kDa
PCRRHMEASLQEFKASPRMVPRAV-----YLPNCDRKGFYKRKQQCKPSRGRKRGICWCVDKY-GMKLPGMEYVDGDFQCHAFDSSNVE                       252 AA    25.7 kDa
PCRRHDSVLQQLQTE-VF-RGGANGL---YVPNCDLRGFYRKRQQCRSSQGNRRGFCWCVDPM-GQPLPVSPDGQGSSQCSARSSG                          201 AA    28.4 kDa
                                                                                                                         21.5 kDa

          *                  *           *        *    ***                 *                    *
Human IGFBP-1                                        APWQCAPCSAEKLALCPPVSAS------------CSE---VTRSAGCGCCPMCALPLGAACGVATARCARGLSCRALPGEQQPLHALTRGQGAC
Human IGFBP-2                                              EVLFRCRPCTPERLAACGPPTPERLAACGPPPVAPPAAVAAVAGGARMPCAE----LVREPGCGCCSVCARLEGEACGVYTPRCGQGLRCYPHPGSELPLQALVMGETC
Human IGFBP-3                                   GASSGGLGPVVRCEPCDARALAQCAPPPAV--------CAE----LVREPGCGCCLTCALSEGQPCGIYTERCGSGLRCQPSPDEARPLQALLDGRGLC
Human IGFBP-4                                              DEAIHCPPCSEEKLARCRPPVG-----------CEE----LVREPGCGCCATCALGLGMPCGVYTPRCGSGLRCYPPRGVEKPLRTLMHGQGVC
Human IGFBP-5                                              LGSFVHCEPCDEKALSMC-PPSPLG--------C-E----LVKEPGCGCCMTCALAEGQSCGVYTERCAQGLRCLPRQDEEKPLHALLHGRGVC
Human IGFBP-6                                                ALARCPGCGQVQAGC-PGG---------------CVEEDGGSPAEGCAEAEGCLRREGQCGVYTPNCAPGLQCHPPKDDEAPLRALLLGRGRC
```

## 12. Insulin-Like Growth Factor Binding Proteins in the Ovary

```
                                                                                                    Calc. MW
(VQESDASAPHAAEAGSPESPESTETEEELLDNFHLMAPSEEDHSILWDAISTYDGSKALHVTNIKKWKE)                      234 AA  25.3 kDa
(EKRRDAEYGASPEQVADNGDDHSEGGLVENHVDSTMNMLGGGSAGRKPLKSGMKELAVFREKVTEQHRQMGKGGKHHLGLEPKKLRPPART) 289 AA  31.3 kDa
(VNASAVSRLRAYLLPAPPAPGNASEEDRSAGSVESPSVSSTHRVSDPKFHPLHSKIIIKKGHAKDSQRYKVDYESQSTDTQNFSSESKRETEYG) 264 AA  28.7 kDa
(MELAEIEAIQESLQPSDKDEGDHPNSFSPCSAHDRRCLQKHFAKIRDSTSGGKMKVNGAPREDARPVPQG)                     237 AA  26.0 kDa
(LNEKSYREQVKIERDSREHEEPTTSEMAEETYSPKIFRPKHTRISELKAEAVKKDRRKKLTQSKFVGGAENTAHPRIISAPEMRQESEQG) 252 AA  28.6 kDa
(LPARAPAVAEENPKESKPQAGTARPQDVNRRDQQRNPGTSTTPSQPNSAGVQDTEMG)                                  216 AA  22.8 kDa

        *                                           *           * *
PCRIELYRVVESLAKAQETS--GE-E-ISKFYLPNCNKNGFYHSRQCETSMDGEAGLCWCVYPWNGKRIPGSPEIRGDPNCQMYFNVQN
PCQQELDQVLERISTMRLPDERGPLEHLYSLHIPNCDKHGLYNLKQCKMSLNGQRGECWCVNPNTGKLIQGAPTIRGDPECHLFYNEQQEACGVHTQRMQ
PCRREMEDITNHLKFINVLSPRGV-----HIPNCDKKGFYKKKQCRPSKGRKRGFCWCVDKYGQPLPGYTKGKEDVHCYSMQSK
SCQSELHRALERLAASQ--S-RTH-EDLYIIPIPNCDRNGNFHPKQCHPALDGQRGKCWCVDRKTGVKLPGGLEPKGELDCHQLADSFRE
PCRRHMEASLQELKASPRMVPRAV---Y---LPNCDRKGFYKRKQCKPSRGRKRGICWCVDKY-GMKLPGMEYVDGDFQCHTFDSSNVE
PCRRHLDSVLQOLQTEVY---RG-AQTLY---VPNCDHRGFYTRKRQCRSSQGRRGPCWCVDRM-GKSLPGSPDGNGSSSCPTGSSG
```

FIGURE 12.1. Alignment of the amino acid sequences of 6 rat and human IGFBPs. Amino acids are shown in one-letter code, and gaps are inserted to allow maximal homology alignment. Identical residues at the corresponding positions in more than 3 IGFBPs are shown in bold letters. The locations of all the cysteines are marked by asterisks, except for the two additional cysteines (bold and underlined) present only in IGFBP-4. The amino acids that cannot be aligned are grouped in parentheses. Potential Asn-linked glycosylation sites are underlined. The rat IGFBP-1, -2, -3, -4, -5, and -6 sequences are from references 47, 35, 48, 42, 41, and 39, respectively, whereas the human IGFBP-1, -2, -3, -4, -5, and -6 sequences are from references 31, 37, 9, 42, 41, and 39, respectively.

TABLE 12.3. Cellular localization of IGFBP mRNAs in adult rat ovary.

| Tissue | IGFBP-1 | IGFBP-2 | IGFBP-3 | IGFBP-4 | IGFBP-5 | IGFBP-6 |
|---|---|---|---|---|---|---|
| Granulosa cells | | | | | | |
| *Healthy* | | | | | | |
|   Primordial | − | − | − | − | − | − |
|   Primary | − | − | − | − | − | − |
|   Secondary | − | − | − | − | − | − |
|   Tertiary | − | − | − | − | − | − |
|   Dominant | − | − | − | − | − | − |
|   Preovulatory | − | − | − | − | − | − |
| *Atretic* | | | | | | |
|   Preantral | − | − | − | + | + | − |
|   Antral | − | − | − | + | + | − |
| Theca interstitial cells | | | | | | |
|   Secondary | − | + | − | − | − | − |
|   Tertiary | − | + | − | +/− | − | − |
|   Dominant | − | + | − | +/− | − | − |
|   Preovulatory | − | + | − | − | − | − |
|   Atretic | − | + | − | − | − | − |
| Secondary interstitial cells | − | + | − | − | +/− | − |
| Corpora lutea | − | − | + | − | +/− | − |
| Oocyte | − | − | − | − | − | − |
| Theca externa | − | − | − | − | − | + |
| Stroma | − | − | − | − | − | + |
| Smooth muscle | − | − | − | − | − | + |
| Surface epithelium | − | + | − | − | + | − |

*Note:* A − = no positive hybridization signal detectable above the background levels seen in control sections incubated with the appropriate sense cRNA probes; + = strong positive hybridization signal compared to controls; + = positive hybridization signal compared to controls; +/− = a positive, but weak, hybridization signal was observed.

strong in those that were preantral and atretic. A variable signal was detected in some secondary interstitial cells, some corpora lutea, and surface epithelium (44). IGFBP-6 was expressed exclusively in theca externa, stroma, and smooth muscle cells (unpublished observations). The most interesting outcome of this study was the localization of the IGFBP-4 and -5 mRNAs exclusively in granulosa cells of atretic antral and preantral follicles, but not in granulosa cells of healthy follicles. This finding implies roles for IGFBP-4 and -5 in the atretic process.

## Biological Effects of IGFBPs on Granulosa Cells

The effects of purified IGFBPs on granulosa cell function were examined using serum-free cultures of rat granulosa cells obtained from immature, diethylstilbestrol-treated rats (29). Both porcine IGFBP-2 and -3 dose-dependently inhibited FSH-stimulated estradiol and progesterone production, with $EC_{50}$ values of 4.1–7.6 nM for IGFBP-3 and 12.6–12.9 nM for IGFBP-2. The addition of rat IGFBP-4 and -5 to the granulosa cell culture also dose-dependently inhibited the FSH-stimulated production of the two gonadal steroids, with $EC_{50}$ values of 8.0–12.5 nM for IGFBP-4 and 18–20 nM for IGFBP-5. Hence, the biological effects of the IGFBPs on granulosa cell function are mainly inhibitory with a relative order of potency: IGFBP-3 > IGFBP-2 = IGFBP-4 > IGFBP-5.

## Production and Characterization of Rat IGFBP Antisera

To investigate the production of IGFBPs in the ovary, specific antisera to each IGFBP are needed. Toward this goal we have generated rabbit polyclonal antibodies to rat IGFBP-2, -4, -5, and -6 utilizing synthetic peptide fragments of the IGFBPs. Selection of the specific sequences for antibody production was guided by the hydropathy plot of each IGFBP, and the most hydrophilic regions were selected. In some peptide fragments a tyrosine residue was added at either the amino- or carboxyterminal to allow coupling to a carrier protein and labeling with radioactive iodine. Specifically, the following rat IGFBP peptide fragments were synthesized by solid-phase methodology: $[Tyr^{154}]$IGFBP-2(154–171)$NH_2$, $[Tyr^{121}]$ IGFBP-4(110–121)$NH_2$ IGFBP-5(86–106)$NH_2$, $[Tyr^{88}]$IGFBP-6(88–108) $NH_2$. The synthetic peptides were coupled to hen egg white ovalbumin with bis-diazotized benzidine, and the conjugates were used to immunize rabbits (45). A rat IGFBP-3 antiserum was raised in rabbit using the purified native protein (46).

Each of the elicited antisera recognized its respective BP specifically on Western blotting, as shown in Figure 12.2: IGFBP-2 antiserum (Rb-3) recognized a band at 30.5 kd; IGFBP-3 antiserum (Rb-78) stained a very broad band between 42 and 45 kd; IGFBP-4 antiserum (Rb-8) recognized two bands at 28 and 24 kd; IGFBP-5 antiserum (Rb-10) stained a major band at 29 kd and a minor band at 30 kd; and IGFBP-6 antiserum (Rb-11) recognized a band at 26.5 kd.

The molecular sizes of the bands recognized by the IGFBP-2, -5, and -6 antisera fit well with their respective calculated molecular masses of 29.6, 28.4, and 21.5 kd; IGFBP-3 and -4, which have potential Asn-linked glycosylation sites, had bands stained by their respective antisera that appeared larger than their core protein masses of 28.9 and 25.7 kd, respectively, due to glycosylation. There was no detectable crossreactivity between the different IGFBPs and other antibodies.

## Regulation of IGFBP Production in Cultured Rat Granulosa Cells

The availability of the specific IGFBP antisera allowed us to investigate the production of IGFBPs in cultured rat granulosa cells. In primary

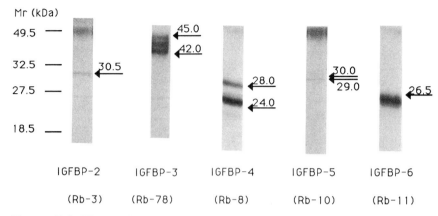

FIGURE 12.2. Western blot of individual rat IGFBPs with the specific antibodies. Fifty nanograms of each IGFBP were loaded onto the gel, followed by SDS-PAGE and immunoblotting with the respective antiserum. In this and subsequent figures, the numbers on the left margin represent the migration positions of the prestained molecular mass standards from Bio-Rad Laboratories, Inc.

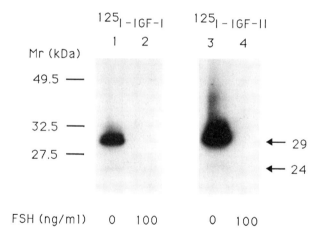

FIGURE 12.3. Ligand blot of the IGFBPs in media of cultured rat granulosa cells treated without (lanes 1 and 3) and with (lanes 2 and 4) 100-ng/mL ovine FSH for 72 h. In the left panel the filter was incubated with [$^{125}$I]IGF-I; in the right panel the filter was incubated with [$^{125}$I]IGF-II.

cultures grown in serum-free medium for 72 h, ligand blotting with [$^{125}$I]-labeled IGF-I and IGF-II revealed two bands migrating at 29 and 24 kd in the media obtained from untreated control cells (Fig. 12.3, lanes 1 and 3), whereas no bands were detectable in media treated with 100-ng/mL FSH

12. Insulin-Like Growth Factor Binding Proteins in the Ovary 161

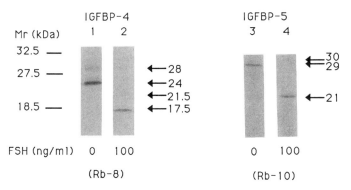

FIGURE 12.4. Identification of the IGFBPs in rat granulosa cell culture media by Western blotting. Lanes 1 and 3 corresponded to media from cells cultured for 72 h without FSH, whereas lanes 2 and 4 were media from cells treated with 100-ng/mL ovine FSH. The IGFBPs in the media were analyzed by Western blotting with the IGFBP-4 antibody Rb-8 (lanes 1 and 2) and the IGFBP-5 antibody Rb-10 (lanes 3 and 4).

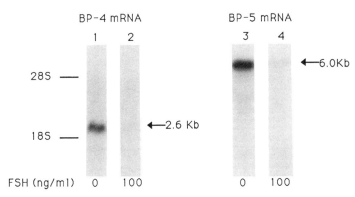

FIGURE 12.5. Identification of IGFBP mRNAs in rat granulosa cells cultured for 72 h in the absence of FSH (lanes 1 and 3) and in the presence of 100-ng/mL ovine FSH (lanes 2 and 4). Ten micrograms of total RNA was loaded onto the gel and, after electrophoresis and transfer to nitrocellulose paper, hybridized with the IGFBP-4 cRNA probe (lanes 1 and 2) and the IGFBP-5 cRNA probe (lanes 3 and 4).

(Fig. 12.3, lanes 2 and 4). Western blotting of the control media with the IGFBP antibodies revealed two bands at 28 and 24 kd with the IGFBP-4 antibody and two bands at 30 and 29 kd with the IGFBP-5 antibody (Fig. 12.4, lanes 1 and 3). By contrast, these bands were absent in media from FSH-treated cells; instead, two lower molecular mass bands of 21.5 and 17.5 kd were detected with the IGFBP-4 antibody, and a 21-kd band was seen with the IGFBP-5 antibody (Fig. 12.4, lanes 2 and 4). This finding suggests that the IGFBP-4 and -5 in the culture media were degraded by an FSH-induced protease. No IGFBPs were detected in the nontreated or FSH-treated media using the IGFBP-2, -3, and -6 antibodies. These results are in accord with the in situ hybridization data that showed that granulosa cells of atretic preantral and antral follicles expressed IGFBP-5 and -4 mRNAs, but not other IGFBP transcripts (43, 44).

To investigate whether expression of the IGFBP-4 and -5 proteins correlates with their mRNAs, we measured the message levels in control and FSH-treated granulosa cells. A single IGFBP-4 mRNA transcript of ~2.6 kb and a 6.0 kb mRNA transcript for IGFBP-5 were detected by Northern blot analysis in control cells (Fig. 12.5, lanes 1 and 3). Treatment with 100-ng/mL FSH caused a marked decrease in the IGFBP-5 mRNA level and total elimination of the IGFBP-4 transcript in the cells (Fig. 12.5, lanes 2 and 4). These findings demonstrate that IGFBP-4 and -5, as well as their mRNAs, are coordinately regulated by FSH in granulosa cells.

## Conclusion

The search for the endogenous FSH-action inhibitor in porcine ovarian follicular fluid led to the identification of five IGFBPs, designated as IGFBP-2, -3, -4, -5, and -6. IGFBP-1 was not found in porcine follicular fluid and rat ovary, even though it was detectable in human follicular fluid. This discrepancy may be explained by species differences in IGFBP expression in the ovary.

Complementary DNAs encoding six IGFBPs have been cloned and their mature protein sequences deduced in rat and human species. Messenger RNAs for IGFBP-2, -3, -4, -5, and -6 were detectable in rat ovary, and each of these mRNAs was found to be expressed in a tissue-specific manner. IGFBP-2 mRNA was expressed in androgen-producing thecal and secondary interstitial cells; the transcript for IGFBP-3 was localized in luteinized granulosa cells; IGFBP-4 and -5 mRNAs were expressed in granulosa cells of atretic antral and preantral follicles; and the IGFBP-6 transcript was localized in the stroma and smooth muscle cells.

One of the major functions of the IGFBPs in the ovary is to block the FSH-stimulated production of gonadal steroids. When rat granulosa cells are removed from their follicles and cultured in serum-free medium, they spontaneously express IGFBP-4 and -5 messages and secrete the two proteins into the culture medium. Coculture of the granulosa cells with FSH (100 ng/mL) inhibits the expression of the IGFBP-4 and -5 genes and also induces the production of a protease that degrades the two IGFBPs. Collectively, these data suggest that IGFBP-4 and -5 may play a role in folliculogenesis. Selection of those follicles that are destined to develop and ovulate could be dependent upon an FSH-rich environment to suppress the expression of IGFBP-4 and -5 in the granulosa cells and to induce the production of a protease to degrade the intrinsic IGFBPs in order to allow the endogenous IGF-I to manifest its synergistic effect with FSH for the promotion of follicle growth and maturation.

*Acknowledgments.* We wish to thank A. Koba, L. Gao, M. Mercado, M. Regno-Lagman, R. Schroeder, and H.-P. Zhang for technical assistance and E. Exum for preparing the manuscript. In addition, we are grateful to the Contraceptive Development Branch of NICHD for providing the porcine follicular fluid and to the National Hormone and Pituitary Program sponsored by NIDDK for providing the ovine FSH. This work was supported by NICHD Contract N01-HD-0-2902 and Program Project Grant HD-09690 from the National Institutes of Health.

## *References*

1. Grady HG, Smith DE. The ovary. Baltimore: Williams and Wilkins, 1962.
2. Richards JS. Maturation of ovarian follicles: actions and interactions of pituitary and ovarian hormones on follicular cell differentiation. Physiol Rev 1980;60:51–89.
3. Erickson GF. An analysis of follicle development and ovum maturation. Semin Reprod Endocrinol 1986;4:233–54.
4. Hsueh AJW, Adashi EY, Jones PB, Welsh TH Jr. Hormonal regulation of the differentiation of cultured ovarian granulosa cells. Endocr Rev 1984;5:76–127.
5. Sluss PM, Reichert LE. Porcine follicular fluid contains several low molecular weight inhibitors of follicle stimulating hormone binding to receptors. Biol Reprod 1984;30:1091–104.
6. diZerega GS, Marrs RP, Roche PC, Campeau JD, Kling OR. Identification of proteins in pooled human follicular fluid which suppress follicular response to gonadotropins. J Clin Endocrinol Metab 1983;56:35–41.
7. Erickson GF, Hsueh AJ. Stimulation of aromatase activity by follicle stimulating hormone in rat granulosa cells in vivo and in vitro. Endocrinology 1978;102:1275–82.
8. Ui M, Shimonaka M, Shimasaki S, Ling N. An insulin-like growth factor-binding protein in ovarian follicular fluid blocks follicle-stimulating hormone-stimulated steroid production by ovarian granulosa cells. Endocrinology 1989;125:912–6.
9. Wood WI, Cachianes G, Henzel WJ, et al. Cloning and expression of the growth hormone-dependent insulin-like growth factor-binding protein. Mol Endocrinol 1988;2:1176–85.
10. Report on the nomenclature of the IGF binding proteins. J Clin Endocrinol Metab 1990;70:817–8.

11. Shimasaki S, Shimonaka M, Ui M, Inouye S, Shibata F, Ling N. Structural characterization of a follicle-stimulating hormone action inhibitor in porcine ovarian follicular fluid; its identification as the insulin-like growth factor-binding protein. J Biol Chem 1990;265:2198–202.
12. Adashi EY, Resnick CE, D'Ercole AJ, Svoboda ME, Van Wyk JJ. Insulin-like growth factors as intraovarian regulators of granulosa cell growth and function. Endocr Rev 1985;6:400–20.
13. Hammond JM, Baranao JLS, Skaleris D, Knight AB, Romanus JA, Rechler MM. Production of insulin-like growth factors by ovarian granulosa cells. Endocrinology 1985;117:2553–5.
14. Oliver JE, Aitman TJ, Powell JF, Wilson CA, Clayton RN. Insulin-like growth factor I gene expression in the rat ovary is confined to the granulosa cells of developing follicles. Endocrinology 1989;124:2671–9.
15. Hernandez ER, Roberts CT Jr, LeRoith D, Adashi EY. Rat ovarian insulin-like growth factor I (IGF-I) gene expression is granulosa cell-selective: 5′-untranslated mRNA variant representation and hormonal regulation. Endocrinology 1989;125:572–4.
16. Adashi EY, Resnick CE, Brodie AMH, Svoboda ME, Van Wyk JJ. Somatomedin-C-mediated potentiation of follicle-stimulating hormone-induced aromatase activity of cultured rat granulosa cells. Endocrinology 1985;117:2313–20.
17. Adashi EY, Resnick CE, Svoboda ME, Van Wyk JJ. Somatomedin-C synergizes with follicle-stimulating hormone in the acquisition of progestin biosynthetic capacity by cultured rat granulosa cells. Endocrinology 1985;116:2135–42.
18. Adashi EY, Resnick CE, Svoboda ME, Van Wyk JJ. Somatomedin-C enhances induction of luteinizing hormone receptors by follicle-stimulating hormone in cultured rat granulosa cells. Endocrinology 1985;116:2369–75.
19. Zhiwen Z, Carson RS, Herington AC, Lee VWK, Burger HG. Follicle stimulating hormone and somatomedin-C stimulate inhibin production of rat granulosa cells in vitro. Endocrinology 1987;120:1633–8.
20. Klein R, Robertson DM, Shukovski L, Findlay JK, de Kretser DM. The radioimmunoassay of follicle-stimulating hormone (FSH)-suppressing protein (FSP): stimulation of bovine granulosa cell FSP secretions by FSH. Endocrinology 1991;128:1048–56.
21. Saito S, Nakamura T, Titani K, Sugino H. Production of activin-binding protein by rat granulosa cells in vitro. Biochem Biophys Res Commun 1991;176:413–22.
22. Cara JG, Rosenfeld RL. Insulin-like growth factor I and insulin potentiate luteinizing hormone-induced androgen synthesis by rat ovarian thecal-interstitial cells. Endocrinology 1988;123:733–9.
23. Magoffin DA, Kurtz KM, Erickson GF. Insulin-like growth factor-I selectively stimulates cholesterol side-chain cleavage expression in ovarian theca-interstitial cells. Mol Endocrinol 1990;4:489–96.
24. Hernandez ER, Resnick CE, Svoboda ME, Van Wyk JJ, Payne DW, Adashi EY. Somatomedin-C/insulin-like growth factor I as an enhancer of androgen biosynthesis by cultured rat ovarian cells. Endocrinology 1988;122:1603–12.
25. Davoren JB, Kasson BG, Li CH, Hsueh AJW. Specific insulin-like growth factor (IGF) I and II binding sites on rat granulosa cells; relation to IGF action. Endocrinology 1986;119:2155–62.

26. Adashi EY, Resnick CE, Hernandez ER, Svoboda ME, Van Wyk JJ. Characterization and regulation of a specific cell membrane receptor for somatomedin-C/insulin-like growth factor I in cultured rat granulosa cells. Endocrinology 1988;122:194–201.
27. Hernandez ER, Hurwitz A, Botero L, et al. Insulin-like growth factor receptor gene expression in the rat ovary: divergent regulation of distinct receptor species. Mol Endocrinol 1991;5:1799–1805.
28. Zhou J, Chin E, Bondy C. Cellular pattern of insulin-like growth factor-I (IGF-I) and IGF-I receptor gene expression in the developing and mature ovarian follicle. Endocrinology 1991;129:3281–8.
29. Bicsak TA, Shimonaka M, Malkowski M, Ling N. Insulin-like growth factor-binding protein (IGF-BP) inhibition of granulosa cell function: effect on cyclic adenosine 3′,5′-monophosphate, deoxyribonucleic acid synthesis, and comparison with the effect of an IGF-I antibody. Endocrinology 1990; 126:2184–9.
30. Lee YL, Hintz RL, James PM, Lee PD, Shively JE, Powell DR. Insulin-like growth factor (IGF) binding protein complementary deoxyribonucleic acid from human HEP G2 hepatoma cells: predicted protein sequence suggests an IGF binding domain different from those of the IGF-I and IGF-II receptors. Mol Endocrinol 1988;2:404–11.
31. Brinkman A, Groffen C, Kortleve DJ, Geurts van Kessel A, Drop SL. Isolation and characterization of a cDNA encoding the low molecular weight insulin-like growth factor binding protein (IBP-1). EMBO J 1988;7:2417–23.
32. Grundmann U, Nerlich C, Bohn H, Rein T. Cloning of cDNA encoding human placental protein 12 (PP12): binding protein for IGF-I and somatomedin. Nucleic Acids Res 1988;16:8711.
33. Brewer MT, Stetler GL, Squires CH, Thompson RC, Busby WH, Clemmons DR. Cloning, characterization, and expression of a human insulin-like growth factor binding protein. Biochem Biophys Res Commun 1988;152:1289–97.
34. Julkunen M, Koistinen R, Aalto-Setälä K, Seppälä M, Jänne OA, Kontula K. Primary structure of human insulin-like growth factor-binding protein/placental protein 12 and tissue-specific expression of its mRNA. FEBS Lett 1988;236:295–302.
35. Brown AL, Chiariotti L, Orlowski CC, et al. Nucleotide sequence and expression of a cDNA clone encoding a fetal rat binding protein for insulin-like growth factors. J Biol Chem 1989;264:5148–54.
36. Margot JB, Binkert C, Mary J-L, Landwehr J, Heinrich G, Schwander J. A low molecular weight insulin-like growth factor binding protein from rat: cDNA cloning and tissue distribution of its messenger RNA. Mol Endocrinol 1989;3:1053–60.
37. Binkert C, Landwehr J, Mary J-L, Schwander J, Heinrich G. Cloning, sequence analysis and expression of a cDNA encoding a novel insulin-like growth factor binding protein (IGFBP-2). EMBO J 1989;8:2497–502.
38. Seppälä M, Wahlström T, Koskimies AI, et al. Human preovulatory follicular fluid, luteinized cells of hyperstimulated preovulatory follicles, and corpus luteum contain placental protein 12. J Clin Endocrinol Metab 1984;58:505–10.
39. Shimasaki S, Gao L, Shimonaka M, Ling N. Isolation and molecular cloning of insulin-like growth factor binding protein-6. Mol Endocrinol 1991;5:938–48.

40. Report on the nomenclature of the IGF binding proteins. J Clin Endocrinol Metab 1992;74:1215–6.
41. Shimasaki S, Shimonaka M, Zhang HP, Ling N. Identification of five different insulin-like growth factor binding proteins (IGFBPs) from adult rat serum and molecular cloning of a novel IGFBP-5 in rat and human. J Biol Chem 1991;266:10646–53.
42. Shimasaki S, Uchiyama F, Shimonaka M, Ling N. Molecular cloning of the cDNAs encoding a novel insulin-like growth factor-binding protein from rat and human. Mol Endocrinol 1990;4:1451–8.
43. Nakatani A, Shimasaki S, Erickson GF, Ling N. Tissue specific expression of four insulin-like growth factor binding proteins (1, 2, 3 and 4) in the rat ovary. Endocrinology 1991;129:1521–9.
44. Erickson GF, Nakatani A, Ling N, Shimasaki S. Localization of insulin-like growth factor-binding protein-5 messenger ribonucleic acid in rat ovaries during the estrous cycle. Endocrinology 1992;130:1867–78.
45. Benoit R, Ling N, Brazeau P, Lavielle S, Guillemin R. Strategies for antibody production and radioimmunoassays. In: Boulton AA, Baker GP, Pittman QJ, eds. Neuromethods; vol. 6. Clifton, NJ: Humana Press, 1987:43–72.
46. Bicsak TA, Nakatani A, Shimonaka M, Malkowski M, Ling N. Insulin-like growth factor binding protein measurement: sodium dodecyl sulfate-stable complexes with insulin-like growth factor in serum prevent accurate assessment of total binding protein content by ligand blotting. Anal Biochem 1990;191:75–9.
47. Murphy LJ, Seneviratne C, Ballejo G, Croze F, Kennedy TG. Identification and characterization of a rat decidual insulin-like growth factor-binding protein complementary DNA. Mol Endocrinol 1990;4:329–36.
48. Shimasaki S, Koba A, Mercado M, Shimonaka M, Ling N. Complementary DNA structure of the high molecular weight rat insulin-like growth factor binding protein (IGF-BP3) and tissue distribution of its mRNA. Biochem Biophys Res Commun 1989;165:907–12.

# 13

# Luteotropic and Luteolytic Effects of Peptides in the Porcine and Human Corpus Luteum

WOLFGANG WUTTKE, HUBERTUS JARRY, LUTZ PITZEL, EVA DIETRICH, AND SABINE SPIESS

The ovaries of most species studied so far contain numerous regulatory peptides, growth factors, and cytokines (reviewed in 1, 2). Many of these peptides are produced by steroidogenic cells (i.e., granulosa, theca, or luteal cells). In addition, the sympathetic and parasympathetic nerve fibers innervating the ovaries also contain numerous neuropeptides (3, 4), many of which are also produced locally by steroidogenic cells. Only a few of the peptides are secreted into the circulation in amounts that allow systemic effects. Most of them exert autocrine and/or paracrine effects within the ovary. Evidence has accumulated that ovulation, the process of *corpus luteum* (CL) formation, CL function, and spontaneous regression (luteolysis) of the CL are regulated by such autocrine- and paracrine-acting factors (1, 5).

In addition to these peptides, locally produced steroids and prostaglandins also play important roles in regulating the function of the CL. Thus, *estradiol* ($E_2$) was shown to be luteotropic in pig CL (6–8) whereas *prostaglandin* $F_{2\alpha}$ (PGF-2α) inhibited P-secretion from luteal cells (reviewed in 9). In the past we have focused our interest on the effects of some regulatory peptides, primarily *oxytocin* (OXT), and cytokines, particularly *tumor necrosis factor* (TNF), in interacting with locally produced $E_2$ and PGF-2α. To accomplish this we used two principal methods.

First, the effects of these compounds alone or in combination on steroidogenesis—that is, *progesterone* (P), *androstenedione* (A), and $E_2$ production—were tested in porcine luteal monolayer cell cultures (7, 10). This method allows demonstration of the direct effects of these substances on steroid production.

However, since the luteal cells kept under these in vitro situations do not communicate with each other, the indirect effects exerted via paracrine mechanisms cannot be studied. Therefore, we have utilized in the past a second method, a *microdialysis system* (MDS), that allows determination of secretion rates of peptides and steroids in the intact human CL kept under organ culture conditions (11) or from porcine CL in freely moving sows (8, 12). Basically, this MDS functions like an artificial capillary that is implanted in individual CL and that has exteriorized inlets and outlets through which the dialysis medium is pumped. The use of this system was first described by Jarry et al. (13, 14) who used it to determine peptide and steroid secretion from rat adrenal glands. Any substance secreted by the CL diffuses in the dialysis medium and can be measured in the effluent fractions. Furthermore, this method allows local application of substances to be tested within individual CL and determination of the steroidogenic reaction of such treated CL.

From investigation in ruminants it is known that PGF-2α is an important luteolytic signal that originates from the uterus and that appears to inhibit luteal P-secretion (1, 9). Simultaneously, it stimulates luteal OXT secretion, causing further release of PGF-2α from the uterus, thereby amplifying the luteolytic process (15). A similar mechanism may be operant in sows since hysterectomy prevents luteolysis. It was therefore not surprising to observe an inhibitory effect of PGF-2α on porcine luteal cell P-production (Table 13.1). Determination of $E_2$ in the culture media, however, indicated that PGF-2α has a stimulatory effect on the production of this steroid. Qualitatively similar effects were observed when OXT or NPY was added to the culture media (Table 13.1). Since the amounts of $E_2$ produced by the luteal cells are such that they undoubtedly result in high intraluteal concentrations within the intact CL, the effects of $E_2$ on P-production were also tested. Surprisingly, $E_2$ had a powerful stimulatory effect on the P-production of porcine luteal cells (Table 13.1).

Other peptides, such as LHRH, *vasoactive intestinal peptide* (VIP), and *angiotensin II* (AII), were without effects under these cell culture conditions. A third group of substances, the cytokines, particularly TNF and *interleukin-2* (IL-2), proved to be potent inhibitors of basal and gonadotropin-stimulated steroidogenesis; that is, they inhibited basal and gonadotropin-stimulated P- and $E_2$ production of cultured luteal cells (15).

TABLE 13.1. Effects of PGF-2α, OXT, NPY, and $E_2$ on basal steroid production of cultivated porcine luteal cells.

|  | Basal release | PGF-2α $(10^{-7}M)$ | OXT $(10^{-7}M)$ | NPY $(10^{-7}M)$ | $E_2$ $(10^{-7}M)$ |
|---|---|---|---|---|---|
| P | 100 ± 2.8% | 35 ± 4.2%* | 46 ± 6.2%* | 25 ± 4.8%* | 187 ± 14%* |
|  | 100% = 363-ng P/3 × $10^5$ cells × 48 h | | | | |
| $E_2$ | 100 ± 3.4% | 250 ± 12%* | 176 ± 8.3%* | 193 ± 11%* | — |
|  | 100% = 124-pg $E_2$/3 × $10^5$ cells × 48 h | | | | |

*$P < 0.01$ vs. basal.

TABLE 13.2. Effects of TNF (3 nM) and IL-2 (150 U/mL) on basal as well as on hCG-stimulated (6 ng/mL) and $E_2$-stimulated ($10^{-7}$ M) P- and $E_2$ release of cultured porcine luteal cells ($2 \times 10^5$ cells/24 h).

|  | Basal | TNF | IL-2 | $E_2$ | $E_2$ + TNF | hCG | hCG + TNF | hCG + IL-2 |
|---|---|---|---|---|---|---|---|---|
| P | $100 \pm 2.8\%$ $100\% = 206$ ng P/well | $53 \pm 7.2\%^{+}$ | $76 \pm 4.8\%^{+}$ | $180 \pm 14\%^{+}$ | $87 \pm 10\%^{++}$ | $236 \pm 16\%^{+}$ | $138 \pm 9.4\%^{*}$ | $179 \pm 10\%^{*}$ |
| $E_2$ | $100 \pm 3.5\%$ $100\% = 51$ pg/well | $62 \pm 5.1\%^{+}$ | $82 \pm 4.3\%^{+}$ |  |  | $120 \pm 12\%$ | $58 \pm 9.3\%^{*}$ | $78 \pm 4.5\%^{*}$ |

$^{+}$ P < 0.05 vs. basal.
$^{++}$ P < 0.05 vs. $E_2$.
$^{*}$ P < 0.05 vs. hCG.

Furthermore, these cytokines also inhibited $E_2$-stimulated P-secretion. A summary of these results is shown in Table 13.2.

In the following experiments we studied luteal OXT, $E_2$, and P-production in intact and hysterectomized sows. These questions were addressed utilizing the above-described MDS in the freely moving sow. To study the spontaneous secretion rates of OXT, $E_2$, and P during the late luteal phase, MDS was implanted into CL of sows at day 8 or 9 after ovulation. Figure 13.1 shows a spontaneous secretory episode of OXT for

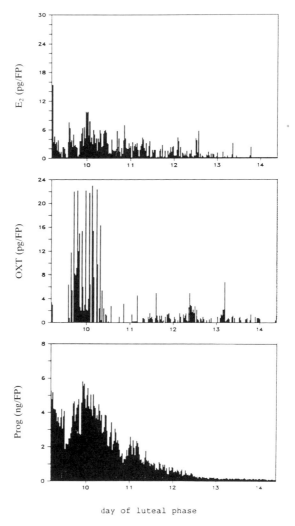

day of luteal phase

FIGURE 13.1. Spontaneous secretion rates of OXT, $E_2$, and P of a porcine CL dialyzed in a freely moving sow prior to and during luteolysis. Note increased OXT release at day 10 that is accompanied by increased $E_2$ and P-release.

an individual CL at the end of day 9 and also shows that this event is accompanied by increased $E_2$ and P-release. Thereafter, the spontaneous secretion rates of the peptide and the two steroids decrease to reach almost undetectable levels between days 12 and 13. This is also the time when P-levels in the serum of the sow are basal, indicating that luteolysis has occurred.

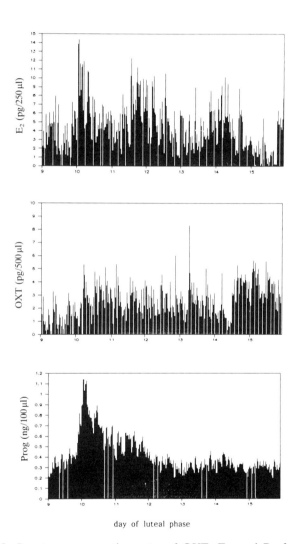

FIGURE 13.2. Spontaneous secretion rates of OXT, $E_2$, and P of a porcine CL dialyzed in a freely moving hysterectomized sow. In comparison to the corresponding secretion rates of CL in a uterus-intact animal (Fig. 13.1), the secretion remained high as a result of the missing uterine luteolytic signal(s).

In contrast to the secretion pattern of these three ovarian hormones, P-levels in dialysates of hysterectomized sows do not decrease (Fig. 13.2), which is in line with published results that porcine CL needs a luteolytic uterine signal. Similarly, OXT and $E_2$ release rates for an individual CL remain at high levels (Fig. 13.2).

What happens when PGF-2α, OXT, or TNF is administered into a CL in which cells are able to communicate with each other? To answer this question, the effects of intraluteal application of PGF-2α and OXT through the MDS were tested in uterus-intact and hysterectomized sows. In earlier experiments we demonstrated that administration of PGF-2α or OXT had a significant stimulatory effect on $E_2$ secretion of young (4–6 days old) CL or luteal cells (8, 16). Hence, they had the same effects as under in vitro cell culture conditions. Surprisingly, in these earlier experiments performed in young CL, OXT was stimulatory to P-secretion, and this effect could be prevented by prior administration of tamoxifen, a specific estrogen receptor blocker (8). This indicated that the direct inhibitory effect of OXT on P-secretion observed under cell culture conditions was overridden by OXT-stimulated $E_2$ secretion that was stimulatory to P-secretion.

In the present study we determined the effects of PGF-2α and OXT in aging CL. Figure 13.3 shows clearly that by day 8 of the luteal phase, OXT was still stimulatory to $E_2$ (Fig. 13.3A) and P- (Fig. 13.3B) secretion. This effect was less pronounced by day 10 and absent in 12- and 14-day-old CL. When OXT was dialyzed in CL of hysterectomized sows, the peptide remained stimulatory to both $E_2$ and P-secretion for the entire investigation period (Figs. 13.4A and 13.4B), which is in contrast to the results obtained in the uterus-intact animals. Qualitatively similar results were obtained when PGF-2α or NPY was dialyzed into CL of uterus-intact or hysterectomized sows (data not shown); that is, these substances were stimulatory to $E_2$ and P-release in hysterectomized sows throughout the time when luteolysis had occurred in uterus-intact animals.

In a recent study it was demonstrated that the number of OXT receptors in young porcine CL was significantly higher than in old CL (17) and that OXT was also less effective in inhibiting P and stimulating $E_2$ secretion in luteal cells obtained from aged CL (16). We concluded, therefore, that OXT serves more luteotropic than luteolytic purposes during the first 10 days of the luteal phase.

The present results indicate further that PGF-2α is also luteotropic in young CL. It is well known that luteolysis in sows depends on a uterine signal that is most likely PGF-2α, as systemic injections of this prostaglandin can induce luteolysis. It is therefore tempting to suggest that OXT and PGF-2α are luteotropic during the first 10 days of the spontaneous cycle. This may also explain why synchronously increased OXT, $E_2$, and P-release are often observed when the spontaneous luteal secretion rates of these hormones are studied (Fig. 13.1). In the absence

13. Effects of Peptides in the Porcine and Human Corpus Luteum 173

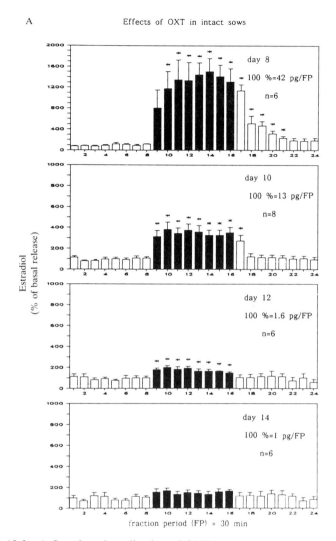

FIGURE 13.3. *A:* Intraluteal application of OXT into porcine CL is stimulatory to $E_2$ secretion by day 8 of the luteal phase. At days 10 and 12, this effect is increasingly less marked and is no longer demonstrable at day 14. The absolute $E_2$ concentrations used to calculate the 100% value are given for each day.

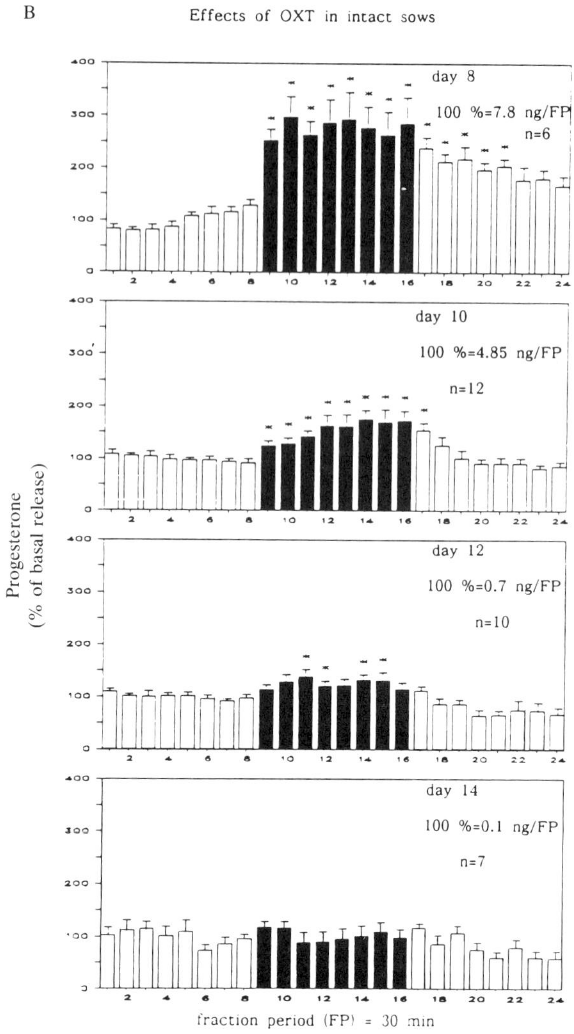

FIGURE 13.3. *Continued. B:* Intraluteal application of OXT into porcine CL is stimulatory to P-secretion only at day 8 of the luteal phase. At days 10 and 12, OXT is less effective and at later days is ineffective in affecting P-secretion. The absolute values used for the 100% calculation are given for each day.

of luteolytic uterine signals—that is, in hysterectomized sows—OXT appears to remain luteotropic due to its maintained stimulatory effect on $E_2$ production. As we have shown above, OXT was never effective in inhibiting luteal P-secretion from the intact CL. As long as it stimulated $E_2$ production, it was also stimulatory to P-secretion. As mentioned earlier, qualitatively similar effects were observed when PGF-2α or NPY was dialyzed into CL.

13. Effects of Peptides in the Porcine and Human Corpus Luteum   175

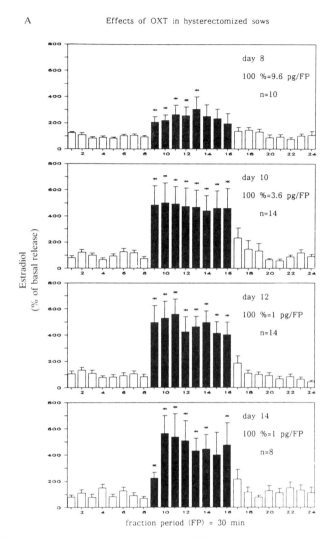

FIGURE 13.4. *A:* Intraluteal application of OXT into CL of hysterectomized sows remains stimulatory to $E_2$ secretion throughout the investigation period. The absolute values are also given. The comparable data of uterus-intact animals are shown in Figure 13.3A.

Hence, there is a large degree of redundant "safety information" operating in the CL. In the case of pregnancy, a trophoblast signal prevents uterine secretion of PGF-2α in the direction toward the ovary (18). This is experimentally mimicked by hysterectomy of our sows and may at least in part explain why hysterectomy prevents luteolysis.

In addition, other mechanisms appear to be involved in the process of

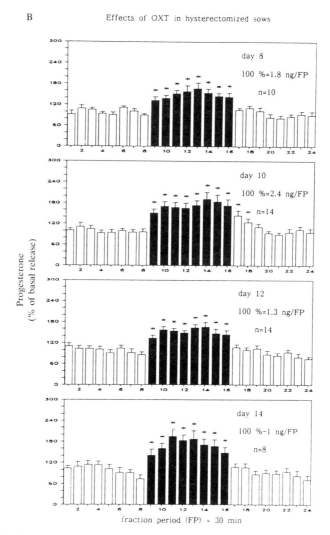

FIGURE 13.4. *Continued. B:* OXT also remains stimulatory to P-secretion. This compares to the data of uterus-intact animals in Figure 13.3B.

luteolysis. As indicated earlier, at the time of luteolysis, macrophages invade the CL (1). On the other hand, it was shown that PGF-2α is a chemoattractant for eosinophils (19), which may suggest that macrophages may also be chemotactically attracted. Macrophages produce cytokines, including TNF.

Finally, TNF was proposed to be involved in the process of luteolysis (15, 20). As shown in our in vitro experiments, TNF not only inhibits P- but also $E_2$ production in cultivated luteal cells. When TNF was dialyzed into CL at days 8, 9, and 10 after ovulation, it had little immediate effect on P-secretion, but the longer the exposure to TNF lasted, the less was the P-output of the CL when compared to the control CL exposed to Ringer solution only. This effect is summarized in Figure 13.5.

Our experimental in vitro and in vivo results suggest, therefore, that the sequence of events during luteolysis may be as follows: A uterine signal, possibly PGF-2α, causes an invasion of macrophages into the aging CL. The TNF produced by these macrophages blocks estradiol production and, therefore, OXT; also, PGF-2α is no longer able to stimulate $E_2$ secretion. Thus, their direct inhibitory effects on P-production add to the direct inhibitory effect of TNF, which results in luteolysis. In the hysterectomized sow the uterine chemoattractant factor does not stimulate macrophage invasion; therefore, OXT and PGF-2α remain luteotropic due to their remaining stimulatory effects on $E_2$ production. We have preliminary evidence that OXT and PGF-2α are indeed luteolytic factors in hysterectomized sows when the CL are preexposed to cytokines, particularly to TNF.

This working hypothesis is schematically shown in Figure 13.6. The luteotropic effects of OXT and PGF-2α are depicted in the upper part of this graph. The deleterious effects of cytokines (particularly of TNF) on the function of CL are detailed in the lower part of this scheme.

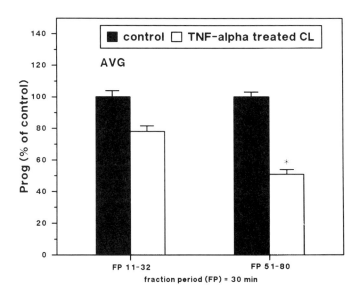

FIGURE 13.5. Mean P-secretion rates of young (days 6–8) porcine CL prior to and during long-lasting (24-h) exposure to TNF (effective intraluteal concentraton: $10^{-10}$M). While P-secretion rates remained high in the control CL, they were significantly reduced in the TNF-exposed CL.

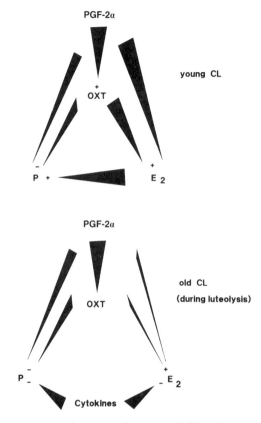

FIGURE 13.6. For an explanation, see "Summary." The thickness of the arrows represents the hypothetical strength of action of the respective paracrine-acting hormone.

## Summary

Our in vitro and in vivo experiments suggest that such substances as PGF-2α and OXT (but possibly also NPY and substance P) have dual effects in porcine CL. They inhibit P-secretion directly, but this effect is counteracted by their stimulatory action on $E_2$ release in the CL. The stimulated $E_2$ production has powerful stimulatory effects in luteal P-secretion. In young CL the net effects of these direct and indirect ($E_2$-mediated) functions are such that $E_2$ dominates; as a result, OXT and PGF-2α are luteotropic (upper part of Fig. 13.6). In aged CL, macrophage products, particularly TNF, inhibit $E_2$ release. As a result, the direct P-inhibitory effects of OXT and PGF-2α become dominant, and their function is therefore luteolytic (lower part of Fig. 13.6).

In addition, TNF also inhibits P-secretion. There is some evidence published that TNF may be produced by rat ovarian steroidogenic cells (21), and we have indications that luteal cells obtained from aged porcine CL have the TNF mRNA. This opens the possibility that nonmacrophage TNF may also be involved in the process of luteolysis.

## *References*

1. Auletta FJ, Flint APF. Mechanisms controlling corpus luteum function in sheep, cows, nonhuman primates, and woman especially in relation to the time of luteolysis. Endocr Rev 1988;9:88–105.
2. Niswender GD, Schwall RH, Fitz TA, Farin CE, Sawyer HR. Regulation of luteal function in domestic ruminants: new concepts. Recent Prog Horm Res 1985;41:101–42.
3. Ojeda SR, Lara H, Ahmed CE. Potential relevance of vasoactive intestinal peptide to ovarian physiology. Semin Reprod Endocrinol 1989;7:52–60.
4. McDonald JK, Dees WL, Ahmed CE, Noe BD, Ojeda SR. Biochemical and immunocytochemical characterization of neuropeptide Y in the immature rat ovary. Endocrinology 1987;120:1703–10.
5. Lamsa JC, Kot SJ, Elderding JA, Nay MG, McCracken JA. Prostaglandin $F_{2\alpha}$-stimulated release of ovarian oxytocin in the sheep in vivo: threshold and dose dependancy. Biol Reprod 1989;40:1215–23.
6. Conley AJ, Ford SP. Direct luteotrophic effect of oestradiol-17β on pig corpora lutea. J Reprod Fertil 1989;87:125–31.
7. Pitzel L, Jarry H, Wuttke W. Effects of oxytocin on in vitro steroid release of midstage small and large porcine luteal cells. Endocrinology 1990;126:2343–9.
8. Jarry H, Einspanier A, Kanngieber L, et al. Release and effects of oxytocin on estradiol and progesterone secretion in porcine corpora lutea as measured by an in vivo microdialysis system. Endocrinology 1990;126:2350–8.
9. Hansel W, Dowd JP. New concept of the control of corpus luteum function. J Reprod Fertil 1986;78:755–68.
10. Pitzel L, Jarry H, Wuttke W. Effects of substance-P and neuropeptide-Y on in vitro steroid release by porcine granulosa and luteal cells. Endocrinology 1991;129:1059–65.
11. Maas S, Jarry H, Teichmann A, Rath W, Kuhn W, Wuttke W. Paracrine actions of oxytocin, prostaglandin $F_{2\alpha}$, and estradiol within the human corpus luteum. J Clin Endocrinol Metab 1992;74:306–12.
12. Einspanier A, Jarry H, Pitzel L, Holtz W, Wuttke W. Determination of secretion rates of estradiol, progesterone, oxytocin, and angiotensin II from tertiary follicles and freshly formed corpora lutea in freely moving sows. Endocrinology 1991;129:3403–9.
13. Jarry H, Düker EM, Wuttke W. Adrenal release of catecholamines and met-enkephalin before and after stress as measured by a novel in vivo dialysis method in the rat. Neurosci Lett 1985;60:273–8.
14. Jarry H, Dietrich M, Düker EM, Wuttke W. Effects of systemic and local administration of etomidate on adrenocortical steroidogenesis in male rats. Acta Endocrinol (Copenh) 1987;114:402–9.

15. Pitzel L, Jarry H, Wuttke W. In the porcine corpus luteum the luteotrophic effects of $PGF_{2\alpha}$ and oxytocin become luteolytic through the action of cytokines. Endocrinology (in press).
16. Pitzel L, Wuttke W. Differential steroidogenic response of porcine small and large luteal cells deriving from young or old corpora lutea. Acta Endocrinol (Copenh) 1990;122:119.
17. Pitzel L, Jarry H, Wuttke W. Demonstration of oxytocin receptors in porcine corpora lutea; comparison of receptor properties in young vs. old corpora lutea. Biol Reprod (in press).
18. Gross TS, Thatcher WW, Hansen PJ, Lacroix MC. Prostaglandin secretion by perifused bovine endometrium: secretion towards the myometrial and luminal sides at day 17 post-estrus as altered by pregnancy. Prostaglandins 1988;35:343–53.
19. Murdoch WJ. Treatment of sheep with prostaglandin $F_{2\alpha}$ enhances production of a luteal chemoattractant for eosinophils. Am J Reprod Immunol Microbiol 1987;15:52.
20. Fairchild-Benyo D, Pate JL. Tumor necrosis factor-α alters bovine luteal cell synthetic capacity and viability. Endocrinology 1992;130:854–60.
21. Sancho-Tello M, Perez-Roger I, Imakawa K, Tilzer L, Terranova PF. Expression of tumor necrosis factor-α in the rat ovary. Endocrinology 1992;130:1359–64.

# 14
# A Role for Neurotrophic Factors in Ovarian Development

SERGIO R. OJEDA, GREGORY A. DISSEN, SASHA MALAMED, AND ANNE N. HIRSHFIELD

In recent years it has become increasingly clear that several growth factors involved in the differentiation of neural cells are similar or identical to those that control the developmental fate of nonneural cells. One of the most striking examples of this regulatory linkage is provided by *stem cell factor* (SCF), the gene product of the mouse *steel* (*Sl*) locus that is required for the differentiation and proliferation of three entirely different cell lineages: neural crest-derived melanocytes, hematopoietic cells, and gonadal germ cells (reviewed in 1). Although SCF induces neither proliferation nor migration of gonadal germ cells, it appears to be essential for their survival (2). Thus, mutations at either the *Sl* locus (that disrupt the synthesis of SCF) or at the *white spotting* (*W*) locus that encodes the SCF receptor (1) severely deplete the number of germ cells able to colonize the genital ridge (2, 3). Strong evidence exists that the SCF receptor is the product of the c-*kit* protooncogene (4), a transmembrane tyrosine kinase receptor encoded by *W* (5).

While activation of the SCF/c-*kit* ligand-receptor complex appears to exert its greatest impact on the early stages of gonadal formation by specifying the number of germ cells that colonize the primitive gonad, recent findings in *Drosophila* have implicated an additional set of *neurogenic* genes in the control of developmental events associated with oogenesis (6). These studies demonstrated that Delta and Notch, two neurogenic genes of the *epidermal growth factor* (EGF) family involved in neuroblast formation, are essential for the differentiation of primordial cells into follicular and follicular-polar cells of the *Drosophila* ovary and are required for specification of the oocyte polarity (6).

In both of the aforementioned examples, the genes involved have various degrees of functional diversity, as they can affect the developmental fate and phenotypic differentiation of a diversity of cell types. Moreover, they are not necessarily produced by their target cells nor do they exert their differentiating influences via chemotropism. These properties have been found to characterize a rapidly growing family of target-derived neurotrophic molecules, of which *nerve growth factor* (NGF) is the most well-characterized member (reviewed in 7).

The NGF gene family currently comprises four members, collectively known as neurotrophins. All of them have been found to be critical for development and survival of neuronal populations in both the peripheral and central nervous systems, but to have different neuronal specificities. The biological actions of neurotrophins are mediated by transmembrane tyrosine kinase receptor molecules encoded by members of the highly related *trk* protooncogene family (8). The *trk* receptors can recognize more than one neurotrophin, but each neurotrophin interacts preferentially with one of the receptors (9). In addition to interacting with the *trk* receptors, all neurotrophins thus far examined bind to another more abundant receptor that lacks tyrosine kinase activity, known as the *low-affinity NGF receptor* (p75 NGF-R) (9). In the case of NGF, evidence exists that the neurotrophin binds to both a *trk* receptor, known as *trk*A, and p75 NGF-R to generate high-affinity binding and effect transmembrane signaling (10).

While the importance of neurotrophins in neuronal development is unquestionable and is currently a subject of intense investigation, recent studies have revealed that neurotrophins and some of their receptors are expressed in a variety of peripheral tissues, with patterns of expression that do not always correlate with the density of innervation (11–17). The presence of key constituents of the neurotrophin molecular complex in nonnervous tissues raises the possibility that neurotrophins are involved in additional, nonneurotrophic functions relevant to the control of developmental and/or differentiating events in the tissues where they are produced (for further discussion, see 18). The ovary offers a particularly useful model to study these novel functions, as it has now been shown to synthesize three of the four known neurotrophins (11, 12, 16, 19) and at least three of the four neurotrophin receptors (13–15, 20). In this chapter we discuss recent findings, including observations derived from a collaborative effort among our laboratories, that suggest a hitherto unsuspected role for ovarian neurotrophins in the control of follicular formation and development.

## Neurotrophins

NGF was the first neurotrophin to be identified and characterized (reviewed in 21, 22). In the central nervous system, NGF is predominantly synthesized in the target fields of magnocellular cholinergic neurons—that is, the hippocampus and the neocortex (23, 24)—and is transported to cholinergic neuronal bodies located in the basal forebrain. Many peripheral tissues innervated by sympathetic and sensory neurons produce NGF that as in the brain is transported in a retrograde fashion by the innervating terminals to the neuronal perikarya, where it exerts its trophic actions (22). The ovary, as a target field of the peripheral sympathetic system (reviewed in 25, 26), is no exception (19).

The biochemical and biological characterization of NGF was greatly facilitated by its abundance in mouse submaxillary gland, a source not available for the other known members of the neurotrophin family. It is not surprising, therefore, that more than 30 years elapsed before a second neurotrophin was characterized and its molecular structure defined (27). This molecule, termed *brain-derived neurotrophic factor* (BDNF), was found to be expressed preferentially in the central nervous system and to promote the survival of several neuronal populations, including cholinergic and dopaminergic neurons of the brain (28, 29). In peripheral tissues, BDNF expression is limited to the heart, lung, and muscle (30), although a recent report showed that BDNF is also produced in fibroblasts, skin, and Schwann cells (31), but not in the ovary (11). The sequence similarity between NGF and BDNF was exploited to isolate and clone another related molecule termed *neurotrophin-3* (NT-3) (30, 32, 33). The expression of NT-3 in brain is much more regionally and developmentally circumscribed than that of BDNF (34, 35). In contrast, NT-3 expression in peripheral tissues is as widespread as that of NGF (11, 30). In the ovary, NT-3 appears to be produced predominantly in granulosa cells of antral secondary and tertiary follicles (11).

These three neurotrophins share approximately 50% of amino acid sequence homology clustered around 6 absolutely conserved cysteine residues that form disulfide bridges essential for proper folding of the protein molecule (reviewed in 7). The resulting three-dimensional configuration has been shown to be required for the biological activity of NGF and BDNF (7) and presumably has the same importance for NT-3.

In experiments in which the evolutionary history of the NGF gene family was reconstructed based on the structural similarities of its members, a fourth neurotrophin termed *neurotrophin-4* (NT-4) was identified by DNA sequence analysis of genomic DNA from *Xenopus* frogs and vipers (12). NT-4 has a 50%–60% amino acid sequence identity with the other members of the family, including strict conservation of the 6 cysteine residues required for spatial configuration. Surprisingly, NT-4 appeared to be expressed only in the *Xenopus* ovary, at levels 100 times greater than those of NGF in heart (12). Although NT-4 promotes neurite outgrowth of sensory neurons of dorsal root ganglia, some of which project to the ovary (36), the exceedingly high levels at which the neurotrophin is expressed in the *Xenopus* ovary suggest that NT-4 is involved in gonadal-specific functions unrelated to its neurotrophic activities (12).

Very recently, an additional member of the neurotrophin family was identified and termed *neurotrophin-5* (NT-5) (16). NT-5 shares about

40%–45% sequence homology with NGF, BDNF, and NT-3 and—in contrast to *Xenopus* NT-4, which does not affect sympathetic neurons—is able to promote the survival of both sensory and sympathetic neurons (16). Its widespread distribution in peripheral tissues is consistent with the interpretation that it serves as a target-derived growth factor for the neurons that innervate these tissues. Evidence has now been provided that NT-5 corresponds to the mammalian counterpart of *Xenopus*/viper NT-4 (17) with which it shares a 64% sequence identity. Mammalian NT-4/NT-5 (henceforth called NT-4) is expressed in the adult rat ovary at low levels, a feature that differs considerably from the strikingly elevated levels of NT-4 found in the *Xenopus* ovary (12), and with the abundant expression of NT-3 in adult rat ovaries (17).

## Neurotrophic Receptors

It has been known for several years that the actions of NGF are initiated by interaction of the peptide with cell-specific membrane-spanning receptor molecules (22). Biochemical studies led to the concept that there are two types of NGF receptors that differ in their relative affinity for NGF. A low-affinity form, called *fast receptor* because of its dissociation constant, comprises the majority (~90%) of the total number of receptors and is expressed in both the nervous system and nonneural tissues (22, 37). The rest (~10%) of the receptors display high-affinity binding for NGF and have been found only in cells responsive to the neurotrophic actions of NGF (22). Interaction of NGF with this high-affinity receptor form is required for the neurotrophin to exert its biological actions.

The low-affinity NGF-R is an ~75-kd glycosylated protein encoded by a single 3.8-kb mRNA species (38, 39). Because of its size, it is also referred to as the p75 NGF-R. It has an extracellular domain that contains the binding recognition sites for NGF (and for the other members of the neurotrophin family as well) and a short intracellular domain that by itself appears unable to mediate signal transduction. Gene transfer experiments involving expression of p75 cDNA revealed that binding of NGF to the p75 receptor alone results in only low-affinity binding and does not lead to measurable biological responses (40). In contrast, expression of p75 in cell lines of neuronal origin known to be responsive to NGF effectively generated high-affinity binding and functional responses. These and other observations led to the concept that formation of NGF high-affinity binding sites requires, in addition to p75, a cell-specific protein(s) that is essential for transmembrane signaling (40 and reviewed in 9). The transmembrane and intracytoplasmic domains of p75 are, however, needed for the formation of the high-affinity receptor complex (41) and receptor-dependent tyrosine phosphorylation events (42).

The identity of the associated protein that participates in the formation of NGF high-affinity binding sites was recently identified as the product of the *trk* protooncogene (43–45). The *trk* receptor (henceforth referred to as *trk*A to distinguish it from the other members of the *trk* gene family) is a tyrosine kinase receptor (46). It has an extensively glycosylated extracellular domain, a single transmembrane domain, and a cytoplasmic domain endowed with a tyrosine kinase catalytic region with sequence homology to other tyrosine kinases (46). Like p75, the *trk*A receptor displays low-affinity binding for NGF (43). Coexpression of both receptors, however, results in high-affinity binding and the initiation of appropriate signal transduction events (10). In addition to NGF, *trk*A recognizes NT-3 (47) and NT-4 (16, 17), but less effectively. It is generally accepted that expression of the *trk*A protooncogene is restricted to the nervous system (48), but this notion may require reevaluation in light of the findings to be described here.

Shortly after the identification of the *trk*A locus, a highly related gene named *trk*B was molecularly characterized (13). The product of this gene is a 145-kd glycoprotein also endowed with tyrosine kinase activity. The *trk*B locus encodes several mRNA species ranging from 9 to 2 kb that, like *trk*A, are preferentially expressed in brain, but also in some peripheral tissues, including lung, muscle, and the adult mouse ovary (13). The presence of *trk*B transcripts in the adult mouse ovary may have developmental and/or functional implications because we have not detected *trk*B mRNA in prepubertal rat ovaries; that is, before the initiation of reproductive cyclicity and corpora lutea formation (Dissen, Ojeda, unpublished observations). Interestingly, the *trk*B locus has also been found to encode a noncatalytic receptor form that lacks most of the cytoplasmic region of the full-size receptor, including the tyrosine kinase domain (49). This *trk*B isoform is preferentially expressed in ependymal cells lining the cerebral ventricles and in the choroid plexus. No information exists regarding the presence of these truncated receptors in nonneural tissues.

The *trk*B receptor recognizes BDNF, NT-3, and NT-4, but not NGF, and mediates functional responses for all three of these neurotrophins (16, 17, 50–52). The magnitude of the biological response mediated by *trk*B is greater when BDNF or NT-4 is employed as ligand, indicating that *trk*B is a preferred BDNF/NT-4 receptor (17, 50–53). Expression of *trk*B in a fibroblast cell line lacking p75 receptors demonstrated that *trk*B is able to mediate BDNF- and NT-3-dependent cell survival and proliferation in the absence of p75 NGF-R (54), suggesting that in contrast to NGF, ligand-induced tyrosine kinase receptor activation is all that is required for effective signal transduction.

Although NT-3 is recognized by *trk*A and *trk*B, the functional consequences of this binding are less conspicuous and/or different than those elicited by NGF and BDNF, respectively (30, 50–52), suggesting the existence of a specific receptor for NT-3. Such a receptor was recently identified as another member of the *trk* tyrosine kinase receptor family and termed *trk*C (14). Transcription of the *trk*C gene results in two mRNA transcripts of 6.1 and 4.7 kb; their translation product is a 145-kd protein that recognizes NT-3, but not NGF or BDNF (14). Expression of the *trk*C gene appears to be restricted to brain tissue, although some evidence exists for the presence of *trk*C mRNA transcripts in the adult rat ovary (14).

These considerations indicate that neurotrophins and their receptors interact in a complex pattern of molecular and cellular specificity that may contribute to the regulation of both neuronal and nonneuronal functions. Differential, tissue-specific level of expression of the neurotrophins, coupled with selective, cell-specific expression of each of their receptors, may prove of importance for the developmental regulation of neuronal survival and the differentiation of specialized nonneuronal cell subsets. A more detailed review of the subject can be found in (7–9) and (55).

# Neurotrophins and Their Receptors in the Developing Mammalian Ovary

## Follicular Development

Because the ovary is innervated by both sympathetic and sensory fibers (reviewed in 25, 26, 56, 57), it would be expected to be a source of target-derived neurotrophic factors. Indeed, both NGF mRNA and its mature protein product have been detected in the immature rat ovary (19), and NT-3 mRNA in the adult ovary as well (11, 17). In experiments performed in one of our laboratories, denervation of the gland of prepubertal rats did not affect NGF mRNA levels, as previously shown in other peripheral tissues (58, 59), but it resulted in increased levels of NGF protein. This is consistent with the concept that target-derived trophic factors are transported in a retrograde fashion by the innervating nerve fibers so that interruption of the transport results in accumulation of the growth factor in the target tissue (60, 61).

To gain insights into the possible influence of the innervation on ovarian development, neonatal rats were injected with polyclonal antibodies to NGF to eliminate peripheral sympathetic neurons (62), and the consequences of this procedure were analyzed several weeks later in peripubertal animals (63). Immunofluorescence procedures revealed an almost complete loss of the ovarian sympathetic innervation. A partial loss of sensory fibers was also detected, mainly as an absence of collateral branching, with relatively intact main fibers. These surviving fibers may derive from sensory neurons that do not need NGF for survival (64). The possibility exists that these neurons are NT-3 responsive because NT-3 supports the survival of NGF-insensitive sensory neurons of the nodose ganglion (30), which contains neurons that project to the ovary (65).

The first ovulation was delayed in immunosympathectomized rats that also exhibited marked irregularities of the estrous cycle. These were characterized by prolonged periods of vaginal acellular profiles interrupted by transient reinitiation of cyclicity, a pattern suggestive of sporadic ovulation. A detailed examination of the neuroendocrine mechanisms underlying these alterations indicated that they most probably result from an ovarian dysfunction. Estradiol release from the ovary in response to gonadotropins was reduced, a deficiency that correlated well with a paucity of large antral follicles in the ovaries of immunosympathectomized rats as compared with age-matched controls (Fig. 14.1). Reflecting the inability of the gland to produce normal amounts of estradiol, plasma LH levels were elevated and LH pulsatility was enhanced in immunosympathectomized animals.

The simplest explanation for these findings is that loss of the innervation caused by blockade of NGF actions during early development of the peripheral sympathetic system removes a facilitatory neural influence on follicular growth. The inability of the immunosympathectomized ovary to interact effectively with the hypothalamic-pituitary unit during the estrous cycle, long after discontinuation of the antibody treatment, also

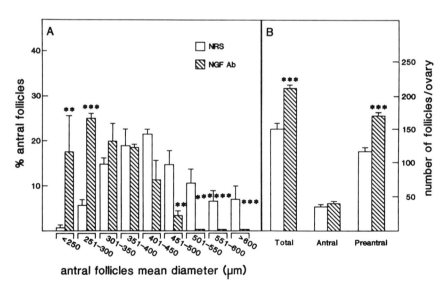

FIGURE 14.1. Effect of neonatal administration of antibodies to NGF (NGF Ab) on follicular development of juvenile rats 29–30 days of age. Morphometric analysis of follicular size was performed as described in reference 63. (**$P < 0.02$; ***$P < 0.001$ vs. NRS-treated controls.) Reprinted with permission from Lara, McDonald, and Ojeda (63), © by The Endocrine Society, 1990.

suggests that ovarian innervation plays a role in amplifying and coordinating the follicular response to gonadotropins. Indeed, clear evidence exists that catecholamines facilitate the effect of gonadotropins on ovarian steroidogenesis (26, 66) and that denervation affects follicular development (25). It is also possible, however, that an additional mechanism responsible for the ovarian dysfunction seen in immunosympathectomized animals is the elimination of a direct influence of neurotrophins on the onset of follicular formation. Experiments addressing this issue are described later in this chapter.

Studies on the response of innervated tissues to nerve injury (67) and on the ontogeny of innervation of peripheral tissues (68, 69) have led to the concept (67) that NGF produced in target tissues binds to p75 NGF-R expressed in nonneuronal cells and that p75, acting as a relay station, transfers the neurotrophin to high-affinity receptors present in the innervating fibers. To have a better understanding of the molecular mechanisms by which NGF may influence the distribution and density of the ovarian innervation, experiments were undertaken to document the presence of p75 NGF-R in the peripubertal ovary and to localize its sites of expression (20). Crosslinking of $^{125}$I-NGF to ovarian membranes followed by immunoprecipitation of the complex and separation of the immunoprecipitated species by SDS-PAGE demonstrated the presence of an ~90-kd protein that corresponds in size to the mature p75 NGF-R bound to a $^{125}$I-NGF monomer (70). That a significant part of these receptors is synthesized in the ovary itself was suggested by the presence of relatively abundant levels of p75 NGF-R mRNA detected by RNA blot hybridization. Interestingly, the steady state levels of p75 NGF-R mRNA changed markedly around the time of first ovulation. The levels that remained elevated between the late juvenile phase (postnatal day 28) and the day of the first preovulatory of gonadotropins decreased abruptly after ovulation. This decline suggested that the receptors are synthesized in developing follicles, but not in corpora lutea. That ovarian expression of the p75 NGF-R gene is not a peculiarity of the rat, but is also manifested in higher primates was indicated by the detection of readily measurable levels of p75 NGF-R mRNA in the ovary of rhesus monkeys (71).

To identify the ovarian cells that express the receptors, the p75 NGF-R protein was localized by immunohistochemistry utilizing a highly specific monoclonal antibody (192 IgG [72]). As expected, the receptor was found in innervating fibers, but to our surprise, thecal cells of developing follicles were strongly immunopositive. Similar findings were made when p75 NGF-R was detected by immunohistochemistry in the prepubertal and adult rhesus monkey ovary (71) and by other authors studying the distribution of p75 NGF-R in various tissues of the adult rat (73).

Examination of the ovary after ovulation revealed the absence of p75 NGF-R immunoreactivity in luteal cells, thus confirming the assumption, made on the basis of Northern blot analysis, that expression of the p75 NGF-R gene is restricted to follicular cells. Not all follicles, however, were immunopositive, and the intensity of the immunoreaction varied considerably among positive follicles. Hybridization histochemistry experiments verified that thecal cells are a major site of p75 NGF-R mRNA expression (Fig. 14.2) and demonstrated that the differences in immunoreactive receptor protein observed previously are, to a significant extent, the consequence of differences in gene expression. In experiments addressed to examine the possibility of a relationship between receptor content and follicular atresia, we found an inverse correlation between the two parameters; that is, a decrease in receptor immunoreactivity as atresia progresses (Dissen, Hirshfield, Ojeda, unpublished observations). Nevertheless, the initial stages of atresia were not accompanied by detectable changes in receptor content, indicating that the loss of p75 NGF-R receptors is a consequence rather than a cause of atresia.

What are the functions of p75 NGF-R in the ovary? Undoubtedly, one of them is to mediate the trophic actions of NGF on the innervation. In considering the previously discussed role of p75 as a relay station, one could envision a process by which NGF (and/or other neurotrophins, such as NT-3) produced in granulosa cells is released to the thecal compartment of the ovary, where it binds to p75 NGF-R. Since these receptors are unable to internalize NGF (22, 37), they may "present" the neurotrophin to the innervating fibers that do express the necessary components for high-affinity binding, namely, the p75 NGF-R and *trk* receptors. Since the size of neuronal target fields is determined by the availability of target-derived neurotrophic factors (7, 69), the extent to which individual follicles are innervated would depend on the level of NGF/NT produced by each follicle and, presumably, on the p75 NGF-R content required to effect the transfer of neurotrophins to the innervating fibers.

A major implication of this concept is that follicular innervation is a dynamic process and that individual follicles are subjected to quantitatively different and changing neural inputs during their life span. The well-established ability of catecholamines and neuropeptides contained in ovarian nerves, such as vasoactive intestinal peptide, to stimulate ovarian steroidogenesis (26, 66) further suggests that the innervation may contribute to the process by which follicular development is regulated and follicles are selected. Figure 14.3 illustrates these concepts. Of interest in this context is the existence of NGF-unresponsive sensory neurons in the neural placode-derived nodose ganglion (74). As indicated before, the nodose ganglion contains perikarya of neurons that project to the ovary (65). Since some of these neurons are sensitive to NT-3 (30) and NT-3 is produced in large antral follicles (11), the possibility exists that NGF and NT-3 act in concert to support the sympathetic and sensory innervation of ovarian follicles. If preferential production of one neurotrophin over the other were to occur in either different follicles or during the life span of a

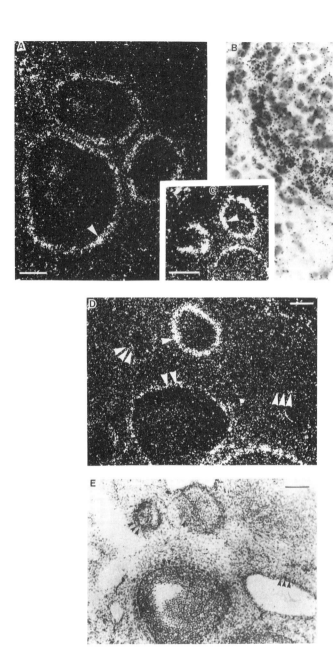

FIGURE 14.2. Identification of p75 NGF-R mRNA in thecal cells (arrowheads) of large antral (*A*) and small follicles (*C*). Panel *B* shows a bright-field view of the localization of p75 NGF-R mRNA in thecal cells of a developing follicle. Expression of p75 NGF-R mRNA varies widely in different follicles (*D* and *E*). Panel *D* shows a dark-field view of different-sized follicles exhibiting a strong, intermediate, or no p75 NGF-R mRNA signal (single, double, and triple arrowheads, respectively). Panel *E* depicts the same area counterstained with thionin. (*A,C,D*, and *E* bars = 100 μM; *B* bar = 20 μM.) Reprinted with permission from Dissen, Hill, Costa, Ma, and Ojeda (20).

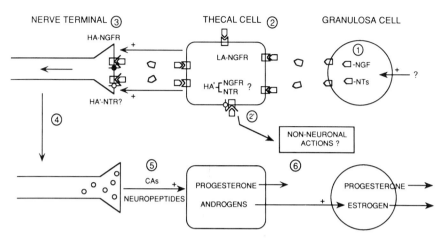

FIGURE 14.3. Hypothetical mechanism by which NGF and NTs may regulate the distribution of the follicular sympathetic innervation. NGF (and NTs), probably produced in granulosa cells (1), binds to low-affinity receptors (LA-NGFR) of thecal cells (2) that then transfer them (3) to high-affinity receptors (HA-NGFR and HA'-NTR) in nerve fibers innervating the follicle; NGF and NTs are then transported to the neuronal perikarya where they initiate their trophic actions. NGF and/or NTs may also have nonneurotrophic effects (2') exerted via hypothetical high-affinity receptors (HA'-NGFR/HA-NTR) on thecal (and granulosa) cells. According to this model the availability of NGF/NTs, dictated by the thecal content of LA-NGFR, would determine the degree of follicular innervation (4). Release of catecholamines (CAs) and neuropeptides (such as VIP) from the innervating fibers (5) increases aromatizable androgen production from thecal cells and progesterone (CAs, VIP) and estrogen (VIP) from granulosa cells. Aromatizable androgens are transported to the granulosa cell compartment where they are converted into estrogen (6). CAs also facilitate the effect of gonadotropins on both thecal and granulosa cells. (+ = stimulation.) Reprinted with permission from Ojeda, Dissen, and Junier (95).

given follicle, the composition of the innervation received would be qualitatively affected.

While these actions are consistent with current concepts regarding the biological actions of target-derived neurotrophic factors, the possibility needs to be considered that neurotrophins may act directly on endocrine cells of the ovary to affect either developmental or differentiated processes. In the case of NGF, such direct actions would require the presence of *trk*A receptors in the putative nonneural target cells. Northern blot analysis of ovarian polyadenylated RNA hybridized to a $^{32}$P-labeled antisense RNA probe demonstrated the presence of a single 3.2-kb mRNA species (15) identical in size to that of *trk*A mRNA detected in rat PC12 cells and striatum in which the *trk*A protooncogene is abundantly expressed. Remarkably, *trk*A mRNA levels were undetectable in prepubertal ovaries and after the first ovulation, but increased strikingly on the day of the first proestrus. The identity of *trk*A mRNA was verified by RNAse protection assay, which demonstrated the ability of ovarian RNA to fully protect a 450-nucleotide antisense RNA complementary to the extracellular domain of *trk*A mRNA. This sensitive assay also revealed that *trk*a mRNA is, indeed, found in prepubertal ovaries, but at exceedingly low levels.

The striking increase in *trk*A mRNA levels observed on the afternoon of first proestrus suggests that expression of the *trk*A protooncogene in the ovary is under hormonal control or that, at the very least, is positively regulated by events that occur at the time of the first preovulatory surge of gonadotropins. Administration of *pregnant mare serum gonadotropin* (PMSG) to 26-day-old immature rats to elicit a premature gonadotropin discharge demonstrated that *trk*A mRNA levels increase only in the afternoon of the expected increase in endogenous gonadotropin surge, suggesting that either gonadotropins or events associated with it are responsible for the preovulatory activation of *trk*A gene expression.

In vitro experiments aimed at clarifying this issue demonstrated the ability of hCG to increase *trk*A mRNA levels in ovarian cell dispersates cultured in serum-free medium. In other experiments, we used hybridization histochemistry to localize the cells that synthesize *trk*A at the time of the normal first preovulatory surge of gonadotropins and found *trk*A mRNA to be present in thecal cells of graafian follicles. No detectable levels were observed in either small antral or preantral follicles, indicating that the *trk*A gene in the ovary is expressed in nonneural cells, and— importantly—that activation of the gene is restricted to a very defined developmental window, critical for the initiation of reproductive capacity. That ovarian *trk*A mRNA is indeed translated into its mature protein product was demonstrated by experiments in which the *trk*A protein was immunoprecipitated with an antibody directed against its carboxyterminal region, followed by protein kinase-mediated receptor autophosphorylation and separation of the phosphorylated species by SDS-PAGE. A phosphorylated species of about 140 kd corresponding to the size of *trk*A in PC12 cells was detected, indicating that the ovary does contain an active *trk*A molecule. Immunoprecipitation of this protein did not occur in the presence of the immunizing peptide.

The functions mediated by the *trk*A receptor in preovulatory follicles are currently unknown. The remarkable activation of *trk*A gene expression in thecal cells during the hours preceding follicular rupture and the ability of *trk* receptors to mediate survival and proliferative responses of fibroblasts to neurotrophins (54, 75) suggests a possible role for neurotrophins in the cytodifferentiation process that accompanies ovulation. Clearly, much more research needs to be done to resolve this issue.

An entirely unexpected observation made in the course of related investigations was the presence of a network of NGF-R-positive neurons in the rhesus monkey ovary (71). In infants the neurons were found to be clustered near the medulla of the ovary. At puberty they had spread into the cortex and were seen associated with developing follicles and in the interstitial tissue. Interestingly enough, no neuronal perikarya were detected in senescent ovaries, suggesting that either the neurons die or they no longer express p75 NGF-R. Another potentially significant feature was the apparent association of some of these neurons with preantral follicles, which they appear to target. Though of great interest because of its potential implications in human physiology, the significance that this neuronal network may have for the regulation of primate ovarian function remains unknown.

## *Initiation of Follicular Formation*

Very recent studies have demonstrated that initiation of follicular development in the rat is an explosive phenomenon that occurs shortly after birth (76, 77). While very few, if any, primordial follicles are detected within the first 24 h postpartum, a striking increase occurs within the next 24 h (76, 77). An initial estimation of the number of follicles formed during this period indicated the development of about 500 follicles between 24 and 36 h after birth and more than double this number during the subsequent 12 h (77). These figures must be considered only approximations because of the inherent difficulties of two-dimensional quantitation to estimate precisely the size of a population anisotropically distributed (78), such as that of primordial ovarian follicles. Nevertheless, they illustrate well the dramatic pace of follicular formation at the onset of folliculogenesis.

The factors that control the initiation of mammalian folliculogenesis have not been elucidated, but they are clearly pituitary independent (reviewed in 79–82). Before formation of the first primordial follicles, the embryonic ovary is formed by three main components: germ cells, mesenchymal cells, and epithelial cells (79, 80). The germ cells originate in the yolk sac of the embryo and migrate to the genital ridge in a process facilitated by the survival-promoting activity of SCF (2, 3). Throughout migration the germ cells proliferate so that their number is in the thousands by the time they finish colonizing the primitive gonad (79). In rodents and primates the germ cells enter the first meiotic prophase at about the time when gonadal sex is morphologically established. They remain arrested in the diplotene stage of the first meiotic prophase until near the time of ovulation at puberty.

The epithelial component of the ovary derives from two sources: the celomic epithelium that contributes to the formation of the genital ridge and the mesonephric tubules (wolffian ducts) that give origin to the ovarian rete (79, 80). Breakup of the mesonephric tubules to form the ovarian rete occurs at about embryonic day 15 in the rat (83) or the 15th week of gestation in humans (84). The ovarian rete comprises an extra-ovarian, a connecting, and an intraovarian portion that form a continuum of cell cords and tubules that extend into the ovary, occupying most of the ovarian medulla and extending towards the ovarian cortex (80, 83). The oocytes, either isolated or in clusters, are surrounded by rete cells. It now appears clear that the epithelial cells of the ovarian rete, and not those of the gonadal surface epithelium, are destined to form the follicular granulosa cells (79, 80, 82).

While the association between rete epithelial cells and oocytes is under way (84), mesonephric mesenchymal cells begin an outward migration from the innermost portion of the ovary. As they migrate (and proliferate), they intercalate among the epithelial cells of the gland and form stromal pockets that contain groups of presumptive granulosa cells and many oocytes. The mesenchymal cells in the walls of the stromal pockets appear to migrate towards the oocytes; the pocketlike organization disappears as the walls invaginate, enclosing presumptive granulosa cells and oocytes into discrete primordial follicles. A primordial follicle is recognized when the single layer of flattened granulosa cells surrounding an individual oocyte is enclosed by a basal membrane (82).

Because of the ability of antibodies to NGF administered on the day of birth to delay follicular development (63), we suspected that neurotrophins could be involved in the control of folliculogenesis. Circumstantial evidence suggesting such a role was also provided by the finding of NGF-like immunoreactivity in male germ cells (85) and NT-4 mRNA in *Xenopus* oocytes (12). Immunohistochemical localization of p75 NGF-R during late fetal-perinatal development of the rat ovary revealed that the receptor was most predominantly present in mesenchymal cells. A high level of expression was found throughout the process of stromal pocket formation, organization of primordial follicles, and development of primary follicles (86). Importantly, p75 NGF-R-positive cells were consistently found enclosing primordial follicles. This and the persistence of p75 NGF-R expression in thecal cells of follicles in more advanced developmental stages strongly suggest that thecal cells originate from these p75 NGF-R-positive mesenchymal cells. It also indicates that p75 NGF-R expression may be used as a molecular marker to identify and follow the developmental fate of mesenchymal cells in the embryonic ovary.

The organization of primordial follicles revealed by the presence of p75 NGF-R in mesenchymal cells is highly reminiscent of the formation of kidney nephrons (87). In this case the undifferentiated nephrogenic epithelium is surrounded by mesenchymal cells endowed with p75 NGF-R; interference with receptor synthesis via administration of antisense oligonucleotides resulted in failure of the nephron to form (87). To assess the possibility that follicular formation may require the presence of neurotrophins, neonatal ovaries were removed before the initiation of follicular formation (less than 10 h after birth), explanted in tissue culture, and exposed to affinity-purified antibodies to NGF for 48h (86). After this time the ovaries were serially sectioned at 5 μm and examined for primordial follicles. As previously reported by other investigators (88, 89), control ovaries showed a spontaneous development of primordial follicles. The antibody treatment, on the other hand, resulted in a dramatic reduction in the number of follicles (304 ± 46 in control ovaries vs. 42 ± 11 in NGF antibodies-treated ovaries). Furthermore, the treated ovaries exhibited widespread death of mesenchymal cells. These results indicate

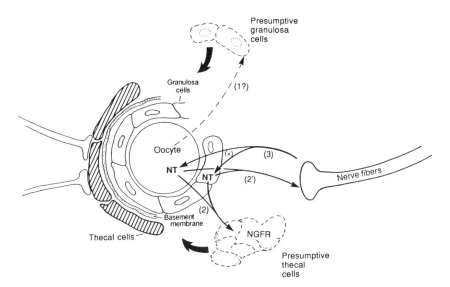

FIGURE 14.4. Hypothetical model for the involvement of neurotrophins in folliculogenesis. Epithelial cells presumably derived from the rete ovary, as described in references 79 and 80, surround diplotene oocytes to become granulosa cells, perhaps as a consequence (1?) of an oocyte-mediated process of lateral induction, as described in reference 96. Either oocytes themselves and/or the surrounding pregranulosa cells produce neurotrophins (NT) that guide the migration of NGF-R-bearing mesenchymal cells towards the pregranulosa cell/oocyte complex (2) and facilitate innervation of the NGF-R-positive, presumptive prethecal cells (2'). Upon reaching their target cells, the innervating fibers cause up-regulation of NT genes (3), as described in references 69 and 68, that in turn enhance expression of NGF-R, as described in reference 97, facilitating completion of follicular formation. The model predicts that the accelerated phase of follicular formation observed in the rat between 24 and 48h after birth, as described in references 76 and 77, is preceded and/or accompanied by an increase in NT and NGF-R synthesis. It also assumes that the effect of the innervation on NT synthesis is, at least in part, neurotransmitter-mediated and that, as such, it becomes evident only when the immature innervating fibers become able to release functionally meaningful amounts of such neurotransmitters. Reprinted with permission from Dissen, Dees, and Ojeda (56).

that neurotrophins play an important role in the initiation of folliculogenesis and suggest that they may be required for survival and proliferation of ovarian mesenchymal cells. Indeed, expression of *trk* genes in differentiated fibroblasts has revealed that neurotrophins can act as survival- and proliferation-promoting factors for these cells (54, 75) and, thus, can effectively mimic the biological actions of fibroblast growth factor.

The gradual organization of p75 NGF-R-positive mesenchymal cells around pregranulosa cells enclosing an oocyte suggests that either the presumptive granulosa cells and/or the oocyte itself produces a diffusible signal that directs the migration of neurotrophin-sensitive cells (Fig. 14.4). Examination of this hypothesis by hybridization histochemical analysis of NGF, NT-3, and NT-4 mRNA expression during the days encompassing the initiation of folliculogenesis revealed an abrupt increase in NT-4 mRNA expression in oocytes on the day of birth; that is, at a time preceding the morphological differentiation of primordial follicles (Dissen, Malamed, Hirshfield, Ojeda, unpublished observations).

These observations suggest that NT-4 plays a fundamental role in the process of mammalian folliculogenesis and that it does so directly via actions exerted on nonneural, endocrine cells of the ovarian follicle. The basic intercellular mechanisms underlying this effect have not been identified. For instance, NT-4 produced in oocytes may attract the presumptive thecal cells by chemotaxis (as a target-derived growth factor would be expected to function). Nevertheless, oocytes are not in direct contact with mesenchymal (thecal) cells and thus cannot be considered as typical target cells. It is also possible that oocytes and the presumptive granulosa cells are reciprocal targets, the interaction of which results in production of a granulosa cell-derived neurotrophin signal that attracts the mesenchymal cells. Figure 14.4 illustrates some of these concepts. Of particular interest in this regard are the observations that the two largest isoforms of the *neural cell adhesion molecules* (NCAM) are expressed in rete ovarii cells (90) and that D*trk*, a *Drosophila* gene encoding a receptor tyrosine kinase highly related to the *trk* family of neurotrophin receptors, has structural homology with NCAM (91). Conceivably then, neurotrophins may contribute to directing the cellular organization of follicles via an intercellular signaling pathway that includes both contact guidance and directional migration (92). Obviously, much work needs to be done to clarify these potential underlying mechanisms.

An additional aspect that requires study concerns the role of the innervation in folliculogenesis. It is clear that the ovarian innervation develops long before the formation of the first primordial follicles (77). Immunohistochemical identification of the early fibers demonstrated that some of them are catecholaminergic, as defined by their content of tyrosine hydroxylase, the rate-limiting enzyme in catecholamine biosynthesis. Interestingly enough, the initial innervation of the rat ovary is limited to the innermost portion of the ovary, a distribution that may have profound physiological implications as this is precisely the region of the gland where follicular formation is initiated (79, 82, 93). In recent experiments we observed that i.p. administration of the neurotoxin 6-hydroxydopamine to newborn rats to eliminate the sympathetic innervation of the ovary resulted in 50% fewer primordial follicles quantitated 48 h later (Malamed et al., unpublished observations). Since the synthesis of NGF has been shown to be induced by either isoproterenol, norepinephrine, or activation of cyclic AMP formation (94), the possibility exists that the sympathetic innervation facilitates follicular formation via neurotransmitter-mediated up-regulation of NGF/NT synthesis (Fig. 14.4).

While much remains to be done, the results thus far obtained indicate that the neurotrophins are not entirely neural specific, but are also important components of key regulatory events affecting the development of the reproductive endocrine system. Because of this and other related considerations (20), we have proposed the term *neuroendocrinotrophic factor* to define these unexpected, but highly specific new functions of neurotrophins (20, 56).

*Acknowledgments.* This work was supported by NIH Grants HD-24870, HD-18185, HD-07438, and HD-27194.

## *References*

1. Witte ON. Steel locus defines new multipotent growth factor. Cell 1990; 63:5–6.
2. Godin I, Deed R, Cooke J, Zsebo K, Dexter M, Wylie CC. Effects of the steel gene product on mouse primordial germ cells in culture. Nature 1991; 352:807–9.
3. Godin I, Wylie C, Heasman J. Genital ridges exert long-range effects on mouse primordial germ cell numbers and direction of migration in culture. Development 1990;108:357–63.
4. Huang E, Nocka K, Beier DR, et al. The hematopoietic growth factor KL is encoded by the *Sl* locus and is the ligand of the c-*kit* receptor, the gene product of the *W* locus. Cell 1990;63:225–33.
5. Chabot B, Stephenson DA, Chapman VM, Besmer P, Bernstein A. The proto-oncogene c-*kit* encoding a transmembrane tyrosine kinase receptor maps to the mouse *W* locus. Nature 1988;335:88–9.
6. Ruohola H, Bremer KA, Baker D, Swedlow JR, Jan LY, Jan YN. Role of neurogenic genes in establishment of follicle cell fate and oocyte polarity during oogenesis in *Drosophila*. Cell 1991;66:433–49.
7. Thoenen H. The changing scene of neurotrophic factors. Trends Neurosci 1991;14:165–70.
8. Barbacid M, Lamballe F, Pulido D, Klein R. The *trk* family of tyrosine protein kinase receptors. Biochim Biophys Acta 1991;1072:115–27.

9. Bothwell M. Keeping track of neurotrophin receptors. Cell 1991;65:915-8.
10. Hempstead BL, Martin-Zanca D, Kaplan DR, Parada LF, Chao MV. High-affinity NGF binding requires coexpression of the *trk* proto-oncogene and the low-affinity NGF receptor. Nature 1991;350:678-83.
11. Ernfors P, Wetmore C, Olson L, Persson H. Identification of cells in rat brain and peripheral tissues expressing mRNA for members of the nerve growth factor family. Neuron 1990;5:511-26.
12. Hallböök F, Ibañez CF, Persson H. Evolutionary studies of the nerve growth factor family reveal a novel member abundantly expressed in *Xenopus* ovary. Neuron 1991;6:845-58.
13. Klein R, Parada LF, Coulier F, Barbacid M. *trk*B, a novel tyrosine protein kinase receptor expressed during mouse neural development. EMBO J 1989; 8:3701-9.
14. Lamballe F, Klein R, Barbacid M. *trk*C, a new member of the *trk* family of tyrosine protein kinases, is a receptor for neurotrophin-3. Cell 1991;66: 967-79.
15. Dissen GA, Hill DF, Ojeda SR. *Trk*A proto-oncogene expression in the developing rat ovary. Prog 74th annu meet Endocr Soc, 1992:58.
16. Berkemeier LR, Winslow JW, Kaplan DR, Nikolics K, Goeddel DV, Rosenthal A. Neurotrophin-5: a novel neurotrophic factor that activates *trk* and *trk*B. Neuron 1991;7:857-66.
17. Ip NY, Ibañez CF, Nye SH, et al. Mammalian neurotrophin-4: structure, chromosomal localization, tissue distribution, and receptor specificity. Proc Natl Acad Sci USA 1992;89:3060-4.
18. Wheeler EF, Bothwell M. Spatiotemporal patterns of expression of NGF and the low-affinity NGF receptor in rat embryos suggest functional roles in tissue morphogenesis and myogenesis. J Neurosci 1992;12:930-45.
19. Lara HE, Hill DF, Katz KH, Ojeda SR. The gene encoding nerve growth factor is expressed in the immature rat ovary: effect of denervation and hormonal treatment. Endocrinology 1990;126:357-63.
20. Dissen GA, Hill DF, Costa ME, Ma YJ, Ojeda SR. Nerve growth factor receptors in the peripubertal rat ovary. Mol Endocrinol 1991;5:1642-50.
21. Levi-Montalcini R. The nerve growth factor 35 years later. Science 1987;237: 1154-62.
22. Green LA, Shooter EM. The nerve growth factor: biochemistry, synthesis, and mechanism of action. Annu Rev Neurosci 1980;3:353-402.
23. Ayer-LeLievre C, Olson C, Ebendal T, Seiger A, Persson H. Expression of the β-nerve growth factor gene in hippocampal neurons. Science 1988;240: 1339-41.
24. Large TH, Bodary SC, Clegg DO, Weskamp G, Otten U, Reichardt LF. Nerve growth factor gene expression in the developing rat brain. Science 1986;234:352-5.
25. Burden HW. The adrenergic innervation of mammalian ovaries. In: Ben-Jonathan N, Bahr JM, Weiner RI, eds. Catecholamines as hormone regulators. New York: Raven Press, 1985:261-78.
26. Ojeda SR, Lara HE. Role of the sympathetic nervous system in the regulation of ovarian function. In: Pirke KM, Wuttke W, Schweiger U, eds. The menstrual cycle and its disorders. Berlin: Springer-Verlag, 1989:26-32.
27. Leibrock J, Lottspeich F, Hohn A, et al. Molecular cloning and expression of brain-derived neurotrophic factor. Nature 1989;341:149-52.

28. Hyman C, Hofer M, Barde Y-A, et al. BDNF is a neurotrophic factor for dopaminergic neurons of the substantia nigra. Nature 1991;350:230–2.
29. Knüsel B, Winslow JW, Rosenthal A, et al. Promotion of central cholinergic and dopaminergic neuron differentiation by brain-derived neurotrophic factor but not neurotrophin 3. Proc Natl Acad Sci USA 1991;88:961–5.
30. Maisonpierre PC, Belluscio L, Squinto S, et al. Neurotrophin-3: a neurotrophic factor related to NGF and BDNF. Science 1990;247:1446–51.
31. Acheson A, Barker PA, Alderson RF, Miller FD, Murphy RA. Detection of brain-derived neurotrophic factor-like activity in fibroblasts and Schwann cells: inhibition by antibodies to NGF. Neuron 1991;7:265–75.
32. Hohn A, Leibrock J, Bailey K, Barde Y-A. Identification and characterization of a novel member of the nerve growth factor/brain-derived neurotrophic factor family. Nature 1990;344:339–41.
33. Rosenthal A, Goeddel DV, Nguyen T, et al. Primary structure and biological activity of a novel human neurotrophic factor. Neuron 1990;4:767–73.
34. Maisonpierre PC, Belluscio L, Friedman B, et al. NT-3, BDNF, and NGF in the developing rat nervous system: parallel as well as reciprocal patterns of expression. Neuron 1990;5:501–9.
35. Phillips HS, Hains JM, Laramee GR, Rosenthal A, Winslow JW. Widespread expression of BDNF but not NT3 by target areas of basal forebrain cholinergic neurons. Science 1990;250:290–4.
36. McNeill DL, Burden HW. Neuropeptides in sensory perikarya projecting to the rat ovary. Am J Anat 1987;179:269–76.
37. Greene LA. The importance of both early and delayed responses in the biological actions of nerve growth factor. Trends Neurosci 1984;7:91–4.
38. Johnson D, Lanahan A, Buck CR, et al. Expression and structure of the human NGF receptor. Cell 1986;47:545–54.
39. Radeke MJ, Misko TP, Hsu C, Herzenberg LA, Shooter EM. Gene transfer and molecular cloning of the rat nerve growth factor receptor. Nature 1987;325:593–7.
40. Hempstead BL, Schleifer LS, Chao MV. Expression of functional nerve growth factor receptors after gene transfer. Science 1989;243:373–5.
41. Hempstead BL, Patil N, Thiel B, Chao MV. Deletion of cytoplasmic sequences of the nerve growth factor receptor leads to loss of high affinity ligand binding. J Biol Chem 1990;265:9595–8.
42. Berg MM, Sternberg DW, Hempstead BL, Chao MV. The low-affinity p75 nerve growth factor (NGF) receptor mediates NGF-induced tyrosine phosphorylation. Proc Natl Acad Sci USA 1991;88:7106–10.
43. Kaplan DR, Hempstead BL, Martin-Zanca D, Chao MV, Parada LF. The *trk* proto-oncogene product: a signal transducing receptor for nerve growth factor. Science 1991;252:554–8.
44. Kaplan DR, Martin-Zanca D, Parada LF. Tyrosine phosphorylation and tyrosine kinase activity of the *trk* proto-oncogene product induced by NGF. Nature 1991;350:158–60.
45. Klein R, Jing S, Nanduri V, O'Rourke E, Barbacid M. The *trk* proto-oncogene encodes a receptor for nerve growth factor. Cell 1991;65:189–97.
46. Martin-Zanca D, Oskam R, Mitra G, Copeland T, Barbacid M. Molecular and biochemical characterization of the human *trk* proto-oncogene. Mol Cell Biol 1989;9:24–33.

47. Cordon-Cardo C, Tapley P, Jing S, et al. The *trk* tyrosine protein kinase mediates the mitogenic properties of nerve growth factor and neurotrophin-3. Cell 1991;66:173–83.
48. Martin-Zanca D, Barbacid M, Parada LF. Expression of the *trk* proto-oncogene is restricted to the sensory cranial and spinal ganglia of neural crest origin in mouse development. Genes Dev 1990;4:683–94.
49. Klein R, Conway D, Parada LF, Barbacid M. The *trk*B tyrosine protein kinase gene codes for a second neurogenic receptor that lacks the catalytic kinase domain. Cell 1990;61:647–6.
50. Squinto SP, Stitt TN, Aldrich TH, et al. *trk*B encodes a functional receptor for brain-derived neurotrophic factor and neurotrophin-3 but not nerve growth factor. Cell 1991;65:885–93.
51. Soppet D, Escandon E, Maragos J, et al. The neurotrophic factors brain-derived neurotrophic factor and neurotrophin-3 are ligands for the *trk*B tyrosine kinase receptor. Cell 1991;65:895–903.
52. Klein R, Nanduri V, Jing S, et al. The *trk*B tyrosine protein kinase is a receptor for brain-derived neurotrophic factor and neurotrophin-3. Cell 1991;66:395–403.
53. Klein R, Lamballe F, Bryant S, Barbacid M. The *trk*B tyrosine protein kinase is a receptor for neurotrophin-4. Neuron 1992;8:947–56.
54. Glass DJ, Nye SH, Hantzopoulos P, et al. *trk*B mediates BDNF/NT-3-dependent survival and proliferation in fibroblasts lacking the low affinity NGF receptor. Cell 1991;66:405–13.
55. Yancopoulos GD, Maisonpierre PC, Ip NY, et al. Neurotrophic factors, their receptors, and the signal transduction pathways they activate. In: Cold Spring Harbor Symposia on Quantitative Biology; vol. LV. Plainview, NY: Cold Spring Harbor Laboratory Press, 1990:371–9.
56. Dissen GA, Dees WL, Ojeda SR. Neural and neurotrophic control of ovarian development. In: Adashi EY, Leung PCK, eds. The ovary. New York: Raven Press, 1992.
57. Ojeda SR, Lara H, Ahmed CE. Potential relevance of vasoactive intestinal peptide to ovarian physiology. Semin Reprod Endocrinol 1989;7:52–60.
58. Roher H, Heumann R, Thoenen H. The synthesis of nerve growth factor (NGF) in developing skin is independent of innervation. Dev Biol 1988;128:240–4.
59. Whittemore SR, Larkfors L, Ebendal T, Holets VR, Ericsson A, Persson H. Increased β-nerve growth factor messenger RNA and protein levels in neonatal rat hippocampus following specific cholinergic lesions. J Neurosci 1987;7:244–51.
60. Korsching S, Thoenen H. Quantitative demonstration of retrograde axonal transport of endogenous nerve growth factor. Neurosci Lett 1983;39:1–4.
61. Palmatier MA, Hartman BK, Johnson EM Jr. Demonstration of retrogradely transported endogenous nerve growth factor in axons of sympathetic neurons. J Neurosci 1984;4:751–6.
62. Levi-Montalcini R, Booker B. Destruction of the sympathetic ganglia in mammals by an antiserum to the nerve-growth promoting factor. Proc Natl Acad Sci USA 1960;42:384–91.
63. Lara HE, McDonald JK, Ojeda SR. Involvement of nerve growth factor in female sexual development. Endocrinology 1990;126:364–75.

64. Barde Y-A. Trophic factors and neuronal survival. Neuron 1989;2:1525–34.
65. Burden HW, Leonard M, Smith CP, Lawrence IE Jr. The sensory innervation of the ovary: a horseradish peroxidase study in the rat. Anat Rec 1983;207:623–7.
66. Hsueh AJW, Adashi EY, Jones PBC, Welsh TH Jr. Hormonal regulation of the differentiation of cultured ovarian granulosa cells. Endocr Rev 1984;5:76–127.
67. Johnson EM Jr, Taniuchi M, DiStefano PS. Expression and possible function of nerve growth factor receptors on Schwann cells. Trends Neurosci 1988;11:299–304.
68. Davies AM, Bandtlow C, Heumann R, Korsching S, Rohrer H, Thoenen H. Timing and site of nerve growth factor synthesis in developing skin in relation to innervation and expression of the receptor. Nature 1987;326:353–8.
69. Wyatt S, Shooter EM, Davies AM. Expression of the NGF receptor gene in sensory neurons and their cutaneous targets prior to and during innervation. Neuron 1990;2:421–7.
70. DiStefano PS, Johnson EM Jr. Identification of a truncated form of the nerve growth factor receptor. Proc Natl Acad Sci USA 1988;85:270–4.
71. Dees WL, Schultea TD, Hiney JK, Dissen G, Ojeda SR. The rhesus monkey ovary contains a developmentally regulated network of nerve growth factor receptor immunoreactive neurons in addition to its extrinsic innervation. Prog 74th annu meet Endocr Soc, 1992:59.
72. Taniuchi M, Johnson EM Jr. Characterization of the binding properties and retrograde axonal transport of a monoclonal antibody directed against the rat nerve growth factor receptor. J Cell Biol 1985;101:1100–6.
73. Amano O, Abe H, Kondo H. Ultrastructural study on a variety of non-neural cells immunoreactive for nerve growth factor receptor in developing rats. Acta Anat (Basel) 1991;141:212–9.
74. Lindsay RM, Thoenen H, Barde Y-A. Placode and neural crest-derived sensory neurons are responsive at early developmental stages to brain-derived neurotrophic factor. Dev Biol 1985;112:319–28.
75. Nye SH, Squinto SP, Glass DJ, et al. K-252a and staurosporine selectively block autophosphorylation of neurotrophin receptors and neurotrophin-mediated responses. Mol Biol Cell 1992;3:677–86.
76. Rajah R, Hirshfield AN. The changing architecture of the rat ovary during the immediate postpartum period: a three dimensional (3D) reconstruction [Abstract]. Biol Reprod 1991;44:152.
77. Malamed S, Gibney JA, Ojeda SR. Ovarian innervation develops before initiation of folliculogenesis. Cell Tissue Res 1992.
78. West MJ, Slomianka L, Gundersen HJG. Unbiased stereological estimation of the total number of neurons in the subdivisions of the rat hippocampus using the optical fractionator. Anat Rec 1991;231:482–97.
79. Byskov AG, Hoyer PE. Embryology of mammalian gonads and ducts. In: Knobil E, Neill J, eds. The physiology of reproduction. New York: Raven Press, 1988:265–302.
80. Byskov AG. Differentiation of mammalian embryonic gonad. Physiol Rev 1986;66:71–117.
81. Peters H. The development of the mouse ovary from birth to maturity. Acta Endocrinol (Copenh) 1969;62:98–116.

82. Hirshfield AN. Development of follicles in the mammalian ovary. Int Rev Cytol 1991;124:43–101.
83. Stein LE, Anderson CH. A qualitative and quantitative study of rete ovarii development in the fetal rat: correlation with the onset of meiosis and follicle cell appearance. Anat Rec 1979;193:197–212.
84. Konishi I, Fujii S, Okamura H, Parmley T, Mori T. Development of interstitial cells and ovigerous cords in the human fetal ovary: an ultrastructural study. J Anat 1986;148:121–35.
85. Olson L, Ayer-LeLievre C, Ebendal T, Seiger A. Nerve growth factor-like immunoreactivities in rodent salivary glands and testis. Cell Tissue Res 1987;248:275–86.
86. Dissen GA, Malamed S, Gibney JA, Hirshfield AN, Costa ME, Ojeda SR. Neurotrophins are required for follicular formation in the mammalian ovary. Soc Neurosci Abstr 1992.
87. Sariola H, Saarma M, Sainio K, et al. Dependence of kidney morphogenesis on the expression of nerve growth factor receptor. Science 1991;254:571–3.
88. Fainstat T. Organ culture of postnatal rat ovaries in chemically defined medium. Fertil Steril 1968;19:317–38.
89. Funkenstein B, Nimrod A, Lindner HR. The development of steroidogenic capability and responsiveness to gonadotropins in cultured neonatal rat ovaries. Endocrinology 1980;106:98–106.
90. Moller CJ, Byskov AG, Roth J, Celis JE, Bock E. NCAM in developing mouse gonads and ducts. Anat Embryol 1991;184:541–8.
91. Pulido D, Campuzano S, Koda T, Modolell J, Barbacid M. D*trk*, a *Drosophila* gene related to the *trk* family of neurotrophin receptors, encodes a novel class of neural cell adhesion molecule. EMBO J 1992;11:391 404.
92. Hynes RO, Lander AD. Contact and adhesive specificities in the associations, migrations, and targeting of cells and axons. Cell 1992;68:303–22.
93. Byskov AG, Lintern-Moore S. Follicle formation in the immature mouse ovary: the role of the rete ovarii. J Anat 1973;116:207–17.
94. Matsuoka I, Meyer M, Thoenen H. Cell-type-specific regulation of nerve growth factor (NGF) synthesis in non-neuronal cells: comparison of Schwann cells with other cell types. J Neurosci 1991;11:3165–77.
95. Ojeda SR, Dissen GA, Junier M-P. Neurotrophic factors and female sexual development. In: Ganong WF, Martini L, eds. Frontiers in neuroendocrinology; vol 13. New York: Raven Press, 1992:120–62.
96. Jessell TM, Melton DA. Diffusible factors in vertebrate embryonic induction. Cell 1992;68:257–70.
97. Miller FD, Mathew TC, Toma JG. Regulation of nerve growth factor receptor gene expression by nerve growth factor in the developing peripheral nervous system. J Cell Biol 1991;112:303–12.

# Author Index

**A**

Albertini, D.F., 79
Allworth, A.E., 79
Atherton-Fessler, S., 60

**B**

Bachvarova, R.F., 25
Besmer, P., 25

**C**

Camaioni, A., 38
Caron-Leslie, L.-A.M., 1
Cidlowski, J.A., 1
Clarke, D.L., 110
Clemens, J.W., 125

**D**

Dean, J., 49
Dietrich, E., 167
Dissen, G.A., 181

**E**

Erickson, G.F., 151

**F**

Fauser, B.C.J.M., 134
Fitzpatrick, S.L., 125

**G**

Griswold, M.D., 100
Guo, Y.-L., 151

**H**

Hascall, V.C., 38
Heckert, L., 100
Hirshfield, A.N., 181
Huang, E.J., 25

**J**

Jarry, H., 167
Ji, I., 89
Ji, T.H., 89

**K**

Koo, Y.B., 89

**L**

Lee, M.S., 60
Ling, N.C., 151
Linzer, D.I.H., 110
Liu, X.-J., 151

**M**

Malamed, S., 181
Malkowski, M., 151
Manova, K., 25
Messinger, S.M., 79
Morris, J.K., 125

**N**

Natraj, U., 125

## O

Ogg, S., 60
Ojeda, S.R., 181

## P

Pache, T.D., 134
Packer, A.I., 25
Parker, L.L., 60
Pitzel, L., 167
Piwnica-Worms, H., 60

## R

Richards, J.A.S., 125

## S

Salustri, A., 38
Schoot, D.C., 134

Shimasaki, S., 151
Sirois, J., 125
Spiess, S., 167

## T

Tirone, E., 38

## W

Wuttke, W., 167

## Y

Yanagishita, M., 38
Young, K.H., 110

# Subject Index

A23187, 6-7, 8-10
N-Acetylglucosamine, 8
Acrosin, 54
Acrosome
  definition, 54
  reaction, 54-55, 57
Actin, 9-10
Actinin (alpha), 10
Actinomycin D, 6-7, 12
Adenosine, 11
Adenylate cyclase, 42, 100
Adenylyl cyclase, 125
Adhesive junctions, 82-84
Adrenal cells, 1, 127, 168
Adrenergic receptors, 101-102
AG18, 129
Agarose, 5, 97, 117-120
AGGTCA motif, 127-128
Allantois, 49
Amino-terminal, 89-90, 92, 96-97, 101-102, 152-154, 155, 159
Ammonium sulfate, 152
AMP. *See* cAMP
Amphibians, oocytes, 82
Androgens, 13, 101, 139-140, 152, 162, 191
Androstenedione, 139, 167
Angiotensin II (AII), 168
Anovulation, 138, 145
Antibodies
  monoclonal, 2, 8-9, 188
  polyclonal, 159, 186-187
Antibody to
  ACK2, 33
  gonadotropins, 25
  c-*kit* ligand, 28-29, 31, 33
  IGFBPs, 159-162
  NGF, 186-187, 194-195
  NGF-R, 188
  p37wee1, 66
  T cell receptor, 4
  TGFB, 46
  *trk*A protein, 192
Antiserum. *See* Antibody
Antrum. *See also* Follicle, antral; Follicle, fluid
  formation of, 38-40, 50, 80
AP-1 transcription factor, 105, 126
AP2 transcription factor, 93-94, 126
AP2E, 92-94
APO-1 epitope, 2
Apoptosis, 1-14, 49
  steroid regulation, 13-14
Apoptotic bodies, 3
Arginine, 70-71
Aromatase, 111, 125-127, 134-135, 139
Asparagine, 155-157, 159
ATP, 2, 9, 112-113, 62-63, 70, 73, 129
Aurintricarboxylic acid (ATA), 4
Autocrine effects, 141, 152, 167
Autodigestion, 7
Autoradiography, 6, 113-114, 118-120
Avidin, 44-45

B cells, 2
Bacteria, cell-cycle regulators, 67-69
Baculoviral expression system, 64-65
Basal membrane, 194-195
BCL2 gene, 13
Benzidine, 159
Biotinylation, 44
Blood, hormones in, 134-135, 137-144
Blot hybridization, 27-28, 160, 188

## Subject Index

Bovine serum, 41–44
Brain, 53, 183, 185–186
Brain-derived neutrophic factor (BDNF), 183–186
Breast tissue, 1, 13
Bryostatin, 129
Buserelin, 143

CAAT box, 127–128
c-Abl protein, 63, 74
*Caenorhabditis elegans*, 1, 12
Calcium
 and apoptosis, 8–11
 channel, 8–9, 13
 FSH and, 100
 intracellular, 8–10, 82, 125, 128
 ionophore, 4, 6–10, 12
 transport, 13, 82
Calf, thymus, 6
Calmodulin, 9–10
cAMP
 analogs, 11
 and apoptosis, 12, 44
 dependent protein kinase, subunit $\beta$ (RII$\beta$), 125–127
 dibutyryl, 41, 44, 46
 FSH and, 41–42, 44, 100, 104
 protein kinase, 73, 128–129
 regulation by, 81–83, 125–127
 synthesis of, 41–42, 44, 96–97, 125, 128–129, 197
cAMP-A-kinase pathway, 128–129
cAMP responsive element (CRE), 92, 127–128
Capacitation, 54, 57
Carboxyterminal, 55, 68–69, 89–90, 101, 110, 112, 154, 155, 159, 192
Carcinogens, 11
Carcinoma, hepatocellular, 61
Cartilage, 39, 44
Casein, 65
Castration, 4
CAT reporter gene, 105–106
Catecholamines, 188–189, 191, 196
CCAAT motif, 51–52, 92, 105
CD3 surface antigen, 9, 11
cdc2$^+$ gene, 64, 67
 gene product, 61, 72

cdc13$^+$ gene, 64
cdc25$^+$ gene, 64, 67–71
 gene product, 63, 67, 69, 72–73
cdc25C gene, 68
 gene product, 65, 67–71
CDC28 gene product, 61
cDNA
 chimeric, 57
 cloned, 89, 91, 94–97, 101, 103–104, 106, 110–111, 152, 154, 162
 for kit-ligand, 27, 33
 for LH receptor, 89, 91, 94–97
 library, 152, 154
 for p75 NGF-R, 184
 for PRL receptor, 110–113, 115
 probes, 103–104
 for zona genes, 52, 55, 57
cdr1+/nim1+ gene, 72
ced3 gene, 12
Cell
 adhesion, 40
 adhesion molecules (CAMs), 82
 death, programmed, 1–14, 49
 lineage, 49
 proliferation, 1, 13, 25–26, 34–35, 50
 volume, 2–3
Cell cycle, 35, 60–74
 cytokinesis, 60
 G1 phase, 60–62
 G2 phase, 60, 62, 72–73, 80
 genes controlling, 63–68, 71–73
 M-phase, 35, 60–62, 72, 74, 79–82
 meiotic, 79–84
 S-phase, 60–61, 73–74
Centrosomes, 80
c-*erb*A, 12
Cerebral ventricles, 185
c-*fos*, 12
Chemotaxis, 196
Chemotherapy, 2, 10, 12
Chemotropism, 182
Chicken, fibroblasts, 129
Chimeras, of zona proteins, 57
Chloramphenicol acetyl transferase (CAT) reporter gene, 105–106
Cholera toxin, 11
Cholesterol side-chain cleavage cytochrome P450, 125–127
Cholinergic neurons, 182–183

## Subject Index

Cholinergic receptors, 101
Chorionic gonadotropin (CG)
  human (hCG), 40–41, 44–45, 141, 143–144, 169, 192
  receptor, 101–102
Choroid plexus, 185
Chromatin, 3–7, 80
Chromatography, 67–68, 152–153
Cis-acting DNA motifs, 128
C-kinase, 9–11, 92, 100, 128–129
c-Ki-ras, 12
c-kit protooncogene, 26–35, 181
Clam, cell cycle regulators, 64
Clomiphene-citrate, 141
Cloning
  cDNA, 57, 101, 103–104, 106, 110–111
  LH receptor cDNA, 89, 91, 94–97
  NT-3, 183
c-myb, 12
c-myc, 12
Coculture, 33
Codon
  start, 106
  stop, 89–90, 94, 96
Coelom, 32
Competence, meiotic, 26, 35, 44, 46, 79–82
Concanavalin A, 12
Contraceptives, oral, 138, 144–145
Coomassie blue, 66, 68
Corpus luteum, 28, 111, 116, 121, 141, 151, 155–158, 167–179, 185, 188
Cortical granules, 54
COS-7 cells, 105–106
Cosmid clones, 89–90
Cotransfection, 93
Cow
  lactogens, 110
  oogenesis, 83
  zona genes, 50
CREB protein, 126–128
cRNA probes, 91–92, 97, 158, 161
Cross-hybridization, nucleic acids, 50
C-Terminal. See Carboxyterminal
Cumulus cells, 38, 41–42, 44, 46, 54, 81–84
  expansion of, 43, 46

Cumulus-oocyte complex (COC), 38, 40, 41, 43–46
  expansion of, 41, 44, 46
Cumulus oophorus, 155
CV-1 cells, 57
Cyclin A, 61–62, 64, 73–74
Cyclin B, 61–64, 69–74
Cyclin-dependent protein kinase (cdk), 61–62, 73–74
Cycloheximide, 11–12
Cysteine, 69, 153–155, 183
Cytochalasin B, 10
Cytochrome P450, 125–127
Cytokines, 167–170, 172, 176–179
Cytokinesis, 60
Cytomegalovirus (CMV) promoter, 57
Cytoplasmic domain, NGF-R, 184–185
Cytoplasmic domain, PRL-R, 110–112, 117–121, 129
Cytoskeleton, 10, 83
Cytotoxicity, 2, 9, 40


Deadenylation, 28, 51–52
Deciduum, 110
Delta gene, 181
Dephosphorylation, 62–63, 65, 69, 71, 73, 81
Depolarization, plasma membrane, 54
Dermatan sulfate proteoglycans (DS-PGs), 39–40, 43–44
Dexamethasone (DEX), 5–6
Diacyl glycerol (DAG), 128
Dialysis, 168, 170–177
Dibutyryl cAMP, 41, 44, 46
Dictyate stage, 50
Diethylstilbestrol, 158
Diplotene stage, 26, 28, 193, 195
Disaccharides, 38
Disulfide bridges, 183
DNA
  binding sites, 51–52
  degradation of, 3–7, 9–11
  injection, 52–53
  internucleosomal, 4–5, 7–9, 11
  protein regulatory units, 128
  sequences, 90–95, 105, 183
  steroid binding, 13
  synthesis of, 60, 63, 73

DNA-protein complex, 52-53
Dog, zona genes, 50
Dopamine receptors, 101-102
Dopaminergic neurons, 183
Dorsal root ganglia, 183
*Drosophila melanogaster*, 181, 196
D*trk* gene, 196


E1A oncogene, 61
E2F transcription factor, 61, 74
*Eco*RI, 90
Electrophoresis, 5-6, 66, 68, 70, 93, 97, 113, 118-120, 160-161, 188, 192
Embryo, 28
  transfer, 142
Endocytosis, 29, 40
Endometrium, 1, 141, 144
Endoplasmic reticulum, 3, 8, 121
Enolase, 65
Eosinophils, 176
Ependymal cells, 185
Epidermal growth factor (EGF), 41-42, 46, 82, 129, 181
  receptor (EGF-R), 129
Epithelium
  ovarian, 193-195
  uterine, 4, 13
ERK1 kinase, 67
ERK2 kinase, 67
Erythrocytes, deficiency, 26
Estradiol, 41, 111, 127, 134-135, 137, 139, 151-152, 158-159, 167-178, 187
Estrogen, 13, 101, 135, 137-139, 141-144, 191
  receptor, 172
Estrous cycle, 151, 187
Ethidium bromide, 5
Exocytosis, 54-55, 57, 83
Exons, 89-90, 94-98, 102-103
  of zona genes, 50-51
Expression vector, 92-93


F9 teratocarcinoma cells, 57
Featherstone, C., 65
Fertilization, 49, 54-55, 57, 79
  in vitro, 138, 141-144

Fibroblast growth factor (FGF), 46, 196
Fibroblasts, 129, 183, 185, 192, 196
Fibronectin, 8
Follicle
  antral, 28, 32, 35, 38-40, 46, 50, 127, 135, 151, 155-158, 162, 183, 187, 189-190, 192
  atresia, 13, 28, 117, 135, 138, 144, 151, 155-158, 162, 189
  developing, 29-34, 40, 46, 50, 134-145, 151, 186-188, 190-197
  dominant, 134-137, 139, 141, 144
  fluid, 38-40, 46, 134-135, 139, 142, 144-145, 151-154, 162
  graafian, 38-39, 41, 44, 192
  innervation of, 186-189, 191-193, 195-197
  NGF-R in, 188-189, 194-195
  nondominant, 136, 138-139, 142
  preantral, 25, 43, 155-158, 162, 187, 192-193
  preovulatory, 125-126, 128-129, 135-136, 142
  primordial, 34, 194-197
  PRL-R synthesis, 116
Follicle cells
  arrest, 33-34, 138-139
  calcium and, 82, 125, 128
  hypertrophy of, 25-26, 33
  proliferation of, 25-26, 34-35, 50
Follicle stimulating hormone (FSH), 40-46, 82, 100-101, 104-105, 111, 125, 127-129, 134-135, 137, 139, 141-144, 151-152, 158-163
  human recombinant, 139, 142
  receptor (FSH-R), 101-104, 151
  receptor (FSH-R) gene, 102-106
  surge, 125, 127-128, 192
Folliculogenesis, 79, 82, 84, 100, 111, 151, 163, 182, 186-188, 193-196
  arrest of, 138-139, 144
Follistatin, 152
Forebrain, 182
Forskolin, 11, 127, 129


G1 phase, 60-62
G1/S transition, 62
G2/M transition, 62-64, 72

## Subject Index

G2 phase, 60, 62–63, 72–73, 80
G-21 protein, 101–102
Galactosamine, 8
Gap junctions, 26, 82–84
Gastrointestinal crypts, 12
Gel filtration, 152–153, 161
Gel retardation assays, 52
Gel shift assay, 93, 127
Gene. *See also* Oncogene; Protooncogene
  activin B, 127–128
  BCL2, 13
  $cdc2^+$, 64, 67
  $cdc13^+$, 64
  $cdc25^+$, 64, 67–71
  cdc25C, 68
  $cdr^+/nim^+$, 72
  ced3, 12
  Delta, 181
  D*trk*, 196
  FSH-R, 102–106
  glutathione S-transferase, 67
  *hsp*70, 12
  inhibin $\alpha$, 127
  LH receptor, 89–90, 92–98, 102–103, 105, 127–128
  luciferase, 53
  $mik1^+$, 72
  milk protein, 110
  NGF-R, 189
  Notch, 181
  $P450_{arom}$, 126–128
  $P450_{scc}$, 126–128
  PGS-2, 127–129
  PR, 127–128
  RII$\beta$, 127–128
  steel (*Sl*), 26–27, 181
  steel panda, 33–34
  *trk*A, 191–192, 196
  *trk*C, 186
  TSH-R, 102–103, 105
  $wee1^+$, 64–68, 71–72
  white spotting (*W*), 26, 34, 181
  Zp2, 50–54
  Zp3, 50–54
Genes. *See also* Promoter; Sequence analysis
  activation of, 35
  apoptosis induction, 12
  dose analyses, 89
  fusion, 105
  homologies, 50–52
  mitotic control, 63–68, 71–73
  NGF family, 181
  oocyte-specific expression, 49, 57
  reporter, 52–53, 105–106
  zona pellucida, 49–54, 57
Genistein, 129
Germ cells, primordial, 26–27, 49
Germinal vesicle breakdown (GVBD), 46, 80, 83
Germinal vesicle stage, 80–81
Gestation. *See* Pregnancy
Gliotoxin, 9, 12
Glucocorticoids, 2, 4, 6–8, 10–13
  receptor, 11
  receptor antagonist, 4–5
Glucosamine, 8
Glutathione, 118, 120
Glutathione agarose, 67–70, 117–119
Glutathione S-transferase (GST), 67–71, 117–118, 120
  gene, 67
Glutathione-S-transferase-PRL-R fusion protein, 117–121
Glycine, 155
Glycosaminoglycans, 38–41, 54
Glycosidases, 54
Glycosylation, 55, 155–157, 159, 184–185
Glycosylphosphatidyl inositol, 39–40
GlyXGlyXXGly sequence, 62
Golgi complex, 80
Gonad, primitive, 49, 181, 193
Gonadal ridge, 32, 49
Gonadotropes, 128
Gonadotropin releasing hormone (GnRH), 128–129
  analogs, 138, 140–143
  receptor, 129
Gonadotropins, 134–135, 139–144, 187–188, 191–192. *See also* specific gonadotropin
  protocol (for IVF), 141–144
  receptors, 127
  regulatory, 38, 40–41
G-proteins, 101–103, 110

Granulosa cells, 100-101, 103, 105, 111, 134, 139, 144, 151-152, 155-163, 167, 183, 189, 191, 194-196. See also Cumulus cells
  and apoptosis, 13
  differentiation of, 125-129
  hyaluronic acid synthesis, 38-39, 43-46
  mural, 38-40, 42, 44-45
  proliferation of, 50
  proteoglycan synthesis, 38-41
  RNA in, 52, 116-117, 121
Growth factor
  epidermal (EGF), 41-42, 46, 82
  fibroblast (FGF), 46
  insulin-like I (IGF-I), 41, 45
  nerve (NGF), 9
  transforming (TGF$\beta$), 12-13, 46
GRP78/BiP, 121

H-7 (PKC inhibitor), 10
Hamster
  zona genes, 50
  zona proteins, 55-57
HC11 mammary cell proteins, 118-121
HCXAGXXR motif, 69
Heart, 183
Heat shock proteins, 121
HeLa cells, 9
Hematopoietic cells, 2, 12, 181
Heparan sulfate proteoglycans (HS-PGs), 39-40
Hepatitis B virus, 61
Hepatocytes, 9
Hexosamine, 38
High-performance liquid chromatography (HPLC), reversed-phase, 152-153
Hippocampus, 182
Hirsutism, 140
Histone H1, 63, 65, 74
  kinase (H1K), 61, 70-71, 81
HL-60 leukemia cells, 12
Homeostasis, 1, 14
Homology, of sequences, 50-52, 55-57, 92, 154-157, 183-184
Hormones. See specific hormone
Hornworm, 12

*hsp*70, 12
Human
  chorionic gonadotropin (hCG), 40-41, 44-45, 96-97, 169, 192
  CG injection (for IVF), 141, 143-144
  corpus luteum, 168
  IGFBPs, 153, 155-157
  ovary, 162
    cell cycle regulators, 61-64, 67-69, 73
    lactogens, 110
    zona genes, 50-53
    zona proteins, 55-57
Hyaluronic acid (HA), 38-39, 41-46
Hybridization, 27, 29, 52, 103, 115-117 152, 155-158, 161-162, 191-192, 196
Hybridomas, 12
Hydropathicity, polypeptides, 56
Hydropathy plot, 159
Hydrophobic regions, 55
6-Hydroxydopamine, 197
17$\alpha$-Hydroxylase, 125-126
Hyperstimulation, ovarian, 141-142, 144
Hypogonadotropic women, 142
Hypophysial luteotrophin, 111
Hypothalamus, 187
Hypothermia, 12
Hysterectomy, 168, 170-172, 174-177


Immune system, 2, 9
Immunoblotting, 159-160
Immunofluorescence, 28, 186
Immunohistochemistry, 28-29, 31, 188-189, 196
Immunoperoxidase, 31
Immunoprecipitation, 66, 188, 192
In vitro fertilization, 138, 141-144
  success rates, 141-142
Indomethacin, 44
Infertility, 138
Inflammation, 2-3
Inhibin, 100, 139, 152
Initiator, 89, 94
Inositol triphosphate (IP3), 9
Insect cells, 69-71
Insulin, 140

Insulin-like growth factor I (IGF-I), 41, 45, 152, 160, 163
 II (IGF-II), 160
 receptors, 154
Insulin-like growth factor binding protein IGFBP-1, 152–158, 162
 IGFBP-2, 152–160, 162
 IGFBP-3, 152–160, 162
 IGFBP-4, 153–163
 IGFBP-5, 153–163
 IGFBP-6, 153–160, 162
Interleukin-1 (IL-1), 10
Interleukin-2 (IL-2), 2, 12–13, 168–170
Interleukin-6 (IL-6), 13
Internucleosome, 4–5, 7–9, 11
Interphase, 80
Interstitial cells, 28–29, 32, 116, 121, 152, 155–158, 162, 193
Intracellular domain, 184–185
Introns, 89, 91, 94, 96–97, 102
 of zona genes, 50–51
Invertebrates, 1, 12, 60–61, 64, 69–71, 81
Iodine, radioactive, 159–160, 188
Ionomycin, 6–8
Ionophore, calcium, 4, 6–10, 12
Isobutylmethylxanthine (IBMX), 81
Isoproterenol, 197


Junctional complexes, 101
Jurkat T cell line, 11


K receptors, 101
Kelley, L.L., 11
Kidney, 53, 194
Kinases, 61–67, 69–74, 80–81, 92, 100, 110–111, 125–129, 181–182, 192, 196
 Kinase A, 126
 Kinase C, 9–11, 92, 100, 128–129
Kinetics, cell cycle, 61
Kyte and Doolittle algorithm, 56


L-929 cells, 57
L19 Ribosomal protein mRNA, 113–114

Lactation, 113–114, 121
Lactogens, placental (PL), 110–111, 114–115
Lamins, 63, 74, 80
Laparoscopy, 134
Lectin, 8
Leucine, 96
Leucine-rich motif, 102–103
Leukemia cells, 2, 10–12
Leydig tumor cells (MLTC), 92
Ligand blot, 160
Lipids, ooplasmic, 82
Liver, 9, 12, 53
 cDNA, 152
 mouse PRL-R, 111–113, 121
 rat, 152
LT/Sv mice, 25
Luc activity, 53
Luciferase, 53, 92–93
Lung, 183, 185
Luteal cells, 111, 125, 144, 167–172, 176, 179, 188
Luteinization, 125–126, 151
Luteinizing hormone (LH), 40–41, 46, 111, 125, 127–129, 140, 142, 151–152, 187
 immunoreactive, 140
 surge, 125–128, 134–136, 192
Luteinizing hormone receptor (LH-R), 89, 101–103, 111, 125, 127, 152
 gene for, 89–90, 92–98, 102–103, 105, 127
Luteolysis, 111, 167–168, 170–172, 175–179
Luteotropic effect, 167, 172, 174, 177–178
Luteotropin, 110–111
Lymphocytes, 9–12
Lymphoma, 4–8, 12, 120–121
Lysine, 71
Lysosomes, 40
Lytic enzymes, 54
Lytic granule, 9


M-phase, 60–62, 72–74, 79–82
M-phase kinase, 80–81
$\alpha_2$-Macroglobulin, 111, 127
Macrophages, 3, 7–9, 12, 176–178

## Subject Index

Macula adherens, 82
Magnesium, 6–8
*Manduca sexta*, 12
Mannosamine, 8
Mast cells, 33
Matrix, extracellular, 41–45, 49–50, 55, 57
Maturation promoting factor (MPF), 61, 63, 81–82
McConkey, D.J., 11
MCK1 kinase, 67
Meiosis. *See also* M-phase; Metaphase
  arrest, 50, 80–83
  cell cycle of, 79–84
  competence for, 26, 35, 44, 46, 79–82
  diplotene stage, 26, 28, 193, 195
  maturation, 49–51, 81
  pachytene stage, 33
  promoting factor (MPF), 35
  prophase, 35, 49–50, 80, 82
  in spermatogonia, 35
Melanocytes, 26, 181
Membrane spanning region. *See* Transmembrane domain
Menstrual cycle, 134–137
  abnormal, 138–140
Mesenchymal cells, 193–196
Mesonephric region, 32, 193–194
Metaphase I, 81
Metaphase II, 79, 81
Microdialysis system (MDS), 168, 170–177
Microfilaments, 10, 83
Microtubules (MT), 80, 83
Microvilli, 3
Mik1$^+$ gene, 72
Milk proteins, 110, 118
Mitochondria, 13
Mitosis. *See also* Cell cycle; M-phase
  activation, 9
  metaphase, 61
  prophase, 80
  yeast, 60–62
Monkey
  CV-1 cells, 57
  ovary, 141, 188, 192–193
Mono Q column, 66
Monoclonal antibodies, 2, 8–9, 188
Moreno, S., 69

Mouse
  gonad development, 49
  granulosa cells, 40
  L-929 cells, 57
  lactogens, 110
  Leydig tumor cells (MLTC), 92
  liver, 111–113, 121
  LT/Sv, 25
  mammary cells, 118–119
  mutants, 26–27, 33–34
  oogenesis, 80–81, 83
  ovary, 111–117, 121, 185
  PRL-R, 111–121
  S49 cells, 4, 7–8, 12
  sterile, 26–27
  submaxillary gland, 183
  thymocytes, 11
  transgenic, 54, 57
  zona genes, 50–54, 57
mRNA for
  calmodulin, 10
  FSH-R, 103–104
  IGFBPs, 155–158, 161–162
  LH-R, 89, 92, 94–98, 125–127
  neurotrophins, 196
  NGF, 186
  NGF-R, 184, 188–190
  NT-3, 186
  NT-4, 194
  PGS, 126, 128
  PR, 126, 128
  PRL-R, 110–117, 121
  p75 NGF-R, 188–190
  TNF, 179
  *trk*A, 191–192
  *trk*B, 185
  *trk*C, 186
  zona genes, 50–52
MSC-1 cells, 105–106
Muscarinic receptors, 101
Muscle, 158, 162, 183, 185
Mutation analysis, 53
Myeloid cells, 13

Natural killer (NK) cells, 2, 9
Nb2 Lymphoma cell proteins, 120–121
Necrosis, 2–4, 9
Nematodes, 1, 12

Neocortex, 182
Nephrons, 194
Nerve growth factor (NGF), 9, 182–189, 191, 196
Nerve growth factor receptor (NGF-R), 182, 188–189, 194–195
 low-affinity (fast), 184–185, 188–189, 191
 gene for, 189
 high-affinity, 184–185, 188, 191
Nerves. See neurons
Nervous system, 182–185
Neural cell adhesion molecules (NCAM), 196
Neural crest, 181
Neuroblast, 181
Neuroendocrinotrophic factor, 197. See also Neurotrophins
Neuromuscular junction, 83
Neurons, 9, 13
 development of, 182
 NGF-R in, 192–193
 parasympathetic, 167
 sensory, 183–184, 186–187, 189
 sympathetic, 167, 183–184, 186–187, 189, 191, 197
Neuropeptides, 167
Neuropeptide VIP, 191
Neuropeptide Y, 168, 172, 174, 178
Neurotoxin, 197
Neurotransmitters, 195, 197
Neurotrophins, 182–189, 191–192, 194–197
Neurotrophin-3 (NT-3), 183–186, 189, 196
Neurotrophin-4 (NT-4), 183–185, 194, 196
Neurotrophin-5 (NT-5), 183–184
Neutrophils, 2, 8
Nifedipine, 9
*p*-Nitrophenyl phosphate (PNPP), 68
Nodose ganglion, 187, 189
Norepinephrine, 197
Northern blot analysis, 52, 91, 94, 97, 103–104, 155, 162, 189, 191
Notch gene, 181
N-Terminal. See Amino-terminal
Nuclear envelope, 3
Nuclease, 4–7, 10, 91, 105
 NUC18, 6–7
Nucleolus, 3, 80
Nucleus, 80
Nurse, P., 69

Obesity, 140
Oct-4 transcription factor, 35
Oligosaccharides, 39, 54
Oncogenes. See also Protooncogenes
 adenoviral E1A, 61
 c-*erb*A, 12
 c-*fos*, 12
 c-Ki-*ras*, 12
 c-*myb*, 12
 c-*myc*, 12
Oocyte
 arrest, 26–27
 atresia, 26, 33
 collection of (IVF), 134, 144
 growth, 25, 30–35, 49, 51, 57, 194
 hyaluronic acid regulation, 39, 43–46
 maturation of, 79–84
 mRNA in, 196
 polarity of, 181
 primordial, 27–28, 33–35, 193–194
Oogenesis, 49–50, 79–83, 100, 181
Oolemma, 54, 83
Orphan receptors, 128
Orthovanadate, sodium, 69–71
Ovalbumin, 159
Ovariectomy, 4
Ovary, 29–32, 49, 89, 100, 103–104, 110–117, 121. See also Cumulus cells; Follicle; Granulosa cells; Mouse, ovary; Rat, ovary; Thecal cells
 apoptosis in, 1
 c-*kit* expression, 27–28
 cDNA in, 152
 *Drosophila*, 181
 epithelium, 193–195
 gene regulation, 126–127, 129
 hyperstimulation of, 141–142, 144
 innervation of, 186–189, 191–193, 195–197
 interstitial tissue, 28–29, 32
 neurotrophins in, 182–184
 NGF-R in, 188
 pig, 38, 152, 162

Ovary (*continued*)
  polycystic, 138-140, 144
  rete, 29, 31-32, 193-196
  RNA in, 191-192
  stroma, 140, 158, 162, 194
  *Xenopus*, 183-184, 194
Oviduct, 41, 49, 54
Ovulation, 41, 44, 49-52, 79-80, 100, 117, 125-126, 128-129, 134-135, 141-142, 151, 167, 170, 187-188, 191-193
  induction of 135, 138-144
Oxytocin, 167-168, 170-178

P11 promoter, 57
$p33^{cdk2}$ kinase, 61-62, 73-74
$p34^{cdc2}$ kinase, 61-65, 67, 69-73, 81
$p37^{wee1}$KD, 66
p75 NGF-R, 182, 184-185, 188-190, 193-194, 196
p80GST-cdc25C, 67-68
p107 protein, 61, 73-74
$p107^{wee1}$ protein, 65, 67, 69-70, 72-73
P450 cytochromes, 125-127
Pachytene stage, 33
PAGE. See Polyacrylamide gel; SDS-PAGE
Palatal shelf tissue, 11
Paracrine effects, 38, 83, 152, 167-168, 178
PC12 cells, 192
Perforin, 9
Perikarya, 189, 191, 193
Perivitelline space, 54, 83
Peroxidase, 44-45
pGEX3X vector, 117
Phagocytosis, 3-4, 7-8
Phenyl Superose, 66
Phorbol esters, 10, 105, 128-129
Phorbol myristate acid (PMA), 128-129
Phosphatase, 63-65, 67-71, 73
Phosphoamino acid analysis, 66-67, 69-70
Phosphodiesterase, 11, 81
  inhibitors of, 41-42
Phospholipase, 10
  C-CA + +-C-kinase pathway, 127
Phospholipids, 8

Phosphorimager, 114
Phosphorus, radioactive, 191
Phosphorylation, 35, 61-63, 65-66, 69-74, 80-81, 128-129, 184, 192
Phosphoserine, 66-67, 69
Phosphothreonine, 62-63, 66
Phosphotyrosine, 62-63, 66-67, 69-72, 81
Pig
  cell culture, 167-169, 172-173, 176
  corpus luteum, 166-178
  hysterectomized, 168, 170-172, 174-177
  IGFBPs, 153, 158
  luteotropic effect, 167, 172, 174
  oocytes, 81
  ovary, 38, 152, 162
  zona genes, 50
Pituitary, 100, 110, 128-129, 142, 151, 187, 193
Placenta, 110, 154
Placental lactogen I (PL-I), 110-111, 114
Placental lactogen II (PL-II), 110-111, 115
Placental phosphatase 1B (PTP1B), 68
Plasma membrane, 3, 7-10, 39-40, 54, 71, 82-83, 101, 110, 151
Plasmid pCAT-basic, 106
Plasmin, 40
Plasminogen activator, 100
Platelet derived growth factor (PDGF) receptor, 26
Polyacrylamide gel, 6, 66, 68, 70, 113, 118-119, 160, 188, 192
Polyadenylation, 94-96, 103, 191
Polyclonal antibodies, 159, 186-187
Polycystic ovary syndrome (PCOS), 138-141, 145
Polymerase chain reaction (PCR), 92, 94, 112-114, 116
Polysaccharides, 38
Polysomes, 28
Polyspermy, 54-55
Posttranscription, 104, 117
Posttranslational modifications, 62
$pp60^{c-src}$ protein, 63, 74
Pregnancy, 49, 110-111, 113-116, 121, 175

rate (IVF), 141-142, 144
Pregnant mare serum gonadotropin (PMSG), 44, 104, 192
Primer extension, 91, 94, 105
Primers, 112-113
Pro-B cells, 13
Proestrus, 192
Progesterone, 13, 41, 111, 128-129, 137, 152, 158-159, 167-174, 176-179, 191
  receptor (PR), 125-128
Prolactin (PRL), 110-111, 114, 121
  receptor (PRL-R), 110-121, 129
Proliferation, of cells, 1, 13, 25-26, 34-35, 50
Prometaphase, 81
Promoter, 52-54, 57, 89, 92-93, 102, 104-106, 110, 127-128
Prophase
  meiotic, 35, 49-50, 80, 82, 193
  mitotic, 80
Prostaglandin E1, 40-41, 44
Prostaglandin E2, 11, 40-41, 44
Prostaglandin endoperoxide synthase (PGS-2), 125-129
Prostaglandin F2a, 167-168, 172, 174-178
Prostaglandin PGF-2a, 111
Prostate gland, 1, 4, 9, 12-13
Protease, 10
  FSH-induced, 162-163
Protein
  binding, 152
  conservation of, 55-56
  kinases. *See* Kinases
  primary structure, 55
  recombinant, 55, 57
  synthesis. *See* Translation
Proteoglycan aggrecan, 39-40
Proteoglycans (PGs), 38-41, 43-44
Proteolysis, 40
Protooncogenes, 12, 26-35, 185
  c-*kit*, 26-35, 181
  *trk*A, 182, 185, 191-192, 196
  *trk*B, 185
  *trk*C, 186
Pseudopregnancy, 94
Puberty, 193

Quin-2, 8

Rabbit
  antibody production, 159
  zona genes, 50
Radioimmunoassay (RIA), 152
Rat
  adrenals, 168
  cell culture, 151, 159-161
  folliculogenesis, 193
  FSH-R, 103-104
  IGFBPs, 153-160
  lactogens, 110
  LH-R gene, 89-92
  ovary, 39-40, 94, 97-98, 128, 154, 155-158, 162, 179, 184-195, 197
  prostate, 9
  serum, 152, 154
  testis, 94
  thymocyte, 7
  zona genes, 50
Reporter genes, 52-53, 105-106
Restriction (R) point, 60
Restriction maps, 89, 106
Rete ovarii, 29, 31-32, 193-196
Retinoblastoma protein, 61
Retinol synchronization, 103-104
Reverse transcription, 112-114, 116
Rhesus monkey, ovary, 188, 192-193
Rhodopsin, 101-102
Ribosomes, 35
Ringer solution, 177
RNA, 52, 113-117, 121. *See also* cRNA; mRNA
  antisense, 191-192
  blots, 27-28
  c-*kit*, 27-28, 30, 33
  probe, 191-192
  synthesis. *See* Transcription
RNAse, 91
RNAse protection assay, 192
Rous sarcoma virus, 129
RU 486, 4-5
Russell, P., 65

S1 nuclease, 91, 105
S49 cells, 4-8, 12

*Saccharomyces cerevisiae*, 61, 67
*Sac*I site, 90
*Schizosaccharomyces japonicus*, 67
*Schizosaccharomyces pombe*, 61, 63–64, 69, 71–73
Schwann cells, 183
SDS-PAGE, 66, 68, 70, 160, 188, 192
Second messenger, 9–10, 42, 82
Seminiferous tubules, 103–104
Sephacryl S-200, 152
Sequence analysis, 33, 64, 90–91, 102, 105, 152–157, 183
Serine, 61–67, 73
Serine/threonine protein kinase, 61–67, 73
Sertoli cells, 26, 100–101, 103–106
Serum. *See* Blood
Sheep, lactogens, 110
Signal
  in cell cycle, 60, 62, 71, 74
  in ovary, 25, 33–34
  peptide, 55
  transduction, 1, 8–13, 54, 83, 110–111, 117, 121, 125–126, 182, 184–185, 196
  uterine, 168, 172, 174, 177
Skin, 183
Solid-phase peptide synthesis, 159
Sonography. *See* Ultrasonography
Sperm, 54–55, 57, 79, 100, 103
Spermatogenesis, 35, 100, 103
Spermiation, 103
S-phase, 60–61, 73–74
SPK1 kinase, 67
Spleen, 53
START point, 60, 62
Steel gene (*Sl*), 26–27, 181
Steel panda gene, 33–34
Stem cell, 13, 53
Stem cell factor (SCF), 181, 193
  receptor, 181
Sterility, mice, 26–27
Steroid hormones. *See also* specific hormone
  and apoptosis, 13–14
Steroidogenesis, 111, 167–168, 188–189
Stroma, 140, 158, 162, 194
STY1/clk1 kinase, 67
Submaxillary gland, 183

Superovulation, 97, 138
SW15, 74


T cells, 2, 9–12
  cytotoxic, 2, 9
  lymphoma, 121
  receptor, 2, 4, 9–10
Tamoxifen, 172
TATA box, 51–52, 89, 92, 105, 126–128
Telophase I, 81
Testes, 13, 35, 53, 94, 100, 103–104
Testosterone, 9, 13, 41, 127, 140
Testosterone-repressed prostate message 2 (TRPM2), 12–13
2,3,7,8-tetra-chlorodibenzo-p-dioxin (TCDD), 9
Thecal cells, 29, 32, 40–41, 125, 152, 155–158, 162, 167, 188–190, 190–192, 194–196
Theophylline, 41
Thionin, 190
3-T-3 cells, 26
Threonine, 61–67, 72–73
Threonine kinase, 73
Thymocytes, 2, 4–13
Thymocytolysis, 11
Thymoma, 12
Thymus, 2, 6, 13, 53
Thyroid stimulating hormone receptor (TSH-R), 101–103
  gene, 102–103, 105
Tissue plasminogen activator (tPA), 125, 128–129
Topoisomerase II, 10
*Trans*-acting factors, 128
Transcription, 97–98, 101, 103–104, 115, 186
  activation of, 110
  apoptosis and, 4, 7
  factors, 35, 53–54, 61, 64, 92–94, 105, 126
  inhibition of, 12
  of kit-ligand, 33
  regulation of, 127–128
  start sites, 89, 91–92, 94, 105–106, 127
  of zona genes, 50–54
Transfection, 96–97, 105, 110

## Subject Index

Transformation, 57, 61
Transforming growth factor B (TGFB), 12, 46
Transgenes, 54, 57, 105
Transglutaminase, 12
Translation, 81, 83, 94, 97, 186, 192
  apoptosis and, 4, 7, 11–12
  of c-*kit*, 28
  inhibitors, 8
  start site, 89–90, 105
Transmembrane domain, 39, 55, 90, 101–103, 110, 112, 117, 181–182, 184–185
Transvaginal ultrasonography, 134–140, 145
Transzonal processes, 83
Triton X-100, 96–97
*trk*A protooncogene, 182, 185, 191–192, 196
  protein, 192
  receptor, 182, 185, 189, 191–192
*trk*B gene, 185
*trk*C gene, 186
Trypan blue, 3
Trypsin, 152
TTTTTAT sequence, 96
Tumor necrosis factor (TNF), 2, 167–170, 172, 176–179
Tyrosine, 62–69, 71–73, 81, 159
Tyrosine hydroxylase, 196
Tyrosine kinase, 54, 62–65, 72–73, 129, 184, 196
  receptor, 26, 181–182, 185–186
Tyrosine phosphatase, 68–69
Tyrphostins, 129

Ultrasonography, 134–140, 144–145
Uterine signals, 168, 172, 174, 177
Uterus, 168, 171–175
  epithelium of, 4, 13

Vaccinia virus, 69

promoter (P11), 57
Valinomycin, 12
Vasoactive intestinal peptide, 168, 189
VH1 phosphatase, 69
Viper, 183–184
Vitronectin, 8


Wee1$^+$ gene, 64–68, 71–72
  gene product, 63–66, 69–70, 72
Western blot, 57, 159–161
White spotting (*W*) gene, 26, 34, 181
Wolffian ducts, 193


*Xenopus laevis*, 63, 183–184, 194
Xyloside (B), 41


Y-chromosome, 49
Yeast
  cell cycle, 60–74
  genes, 63–68, 71–73
Yolk sac, 193
YPK1 kinase, 67


Zona genes, 49–54, 57
  initiation site, 51–53
  promoter region, 52–54
  transcription of, 50–54
Zona pellucida
  chimeric, 57
  definition, 41
  deposition of, 34–35
  function, 49, 54–57, 83
  proteins, 49–50, 54–57
Zona reaction, 54–55
Zp2 gene, 50–54
  protein, 50, 54–57
Zp3 gene, 50–54
  protein, 50, 54–57
  recombinant protein, 55